A Scientist in Wonderland

A Memoir of Searching for Truth
and Finding Trouble

EDZARD ERNST, MD, PhD

imprint-academic.com

Published in the UK by
Imprint Academic, PO Box 200, Exeter EX5 5YX, UK

Distributed in the USA by
Ingram Book Company,
One Ingram Blvd., La Vergne, TN 37086, USA

ISBN 9781845407773

A CIP catalogue record for this book is available from the
British Library and US Library of Congress

To Danielle

Contents

Prelude

There are some people, a fortunate few, who seem to know from an early age where they want to go in life, and have no trouble getting there.

I was not one of them. I was born in Germany in the years immediately following the end of World War II and, like many German children of that era, I was acutely aware of the awkwardness and unease that my elders displayed when it came to discussions that touched on the country's recent history. Even as a young boy, I was conscious that there was a large and restive skeleton in the nation's closet, and that it belonged to all of us—even those of us who had not been alive during the Nazi era were somehow nevertheless its legatees, inextricably bound to it simply by the awareness of its existence.

With time, the growing realization that so many of our peers —teachers, uncles, aunts; perhaps even our own parents—had lent their assent, or worse, their enthusiastic assistance to the Nazi regime robbed their generation of its moral authority and left us, their children, unmoored and adrift.

In a profound sense I felt homeless. An accident of fate had landed me on the planet with a German passport, and with German as my mother tongue, but where did I really belong? Where would I go? What would I do with my life?

There had been physicians in my family for generations and there was always an expectation that I, too, would enter that profession. Yet I felt no strong pull towards medicine. As a young man my only real passion was music, particularly jazz, with its anarchic improvisations and disobedient rhythms; and the fact that it had been banned by the Nazis only made it all the more appealing to me. I would have been perfectly happy to linger indefinitely in the world of music, but eventually, like a debt come due, medicine summoned me, and I surrendered myself to the profession of my forebears.

In hindsight I am glad that my mother nudged me gently yet insistently in the direction of medical school. While music has delighted and comforted me throughout my life, it has been medicine that has truly defined me, stretching, challenging and nourishing me intellectually, even as it tested me on a personal level almost to the limits of my endurance.

Certainly, I had never anticipated that asking basic and necessary questions as a scientist might prove so fiercely controversial, and that as a result of my research I might become involved in ideological wrangling and political intrigue emanating from the highest level.

If I had known the difficulties I would face, the stark choices, the conflicts and machinations that awaited me, would I have chosen to spend my life in medicine? Yes, I would. Becoming a physician and pursuing the career of a scientist have afforded me not only the opportunity to speak out against the dangerous and growing influence of pseudoscience in medicine, but also, paradoxically, it has given me both the reason and the courage to look back steadily at the unbearable past.

This is the story of how I finally found where I belong.

Chapter 1

Early Days

Now that I come to think of it, alternative medicine was always there, all around me. And I was entirely at ease with it. Hydrotherapy, homeopathy, naturopathy—these ideas were as much an accepted and unremarkable part of German life as lederhosen, and perhaps particularly so in Bavaria, which is where I grew up.

No one would therefore have been surprised to see my mother, brother and me stumbling sleepily through the wet grass in front of our house at the crack of dawn, barefoot, and dressed in little more than our underwear. My mother—a most determined and in many ways an endearingly eccentric woman —was an enthusiastic devotee of alternative medicine. For a while she embraced Kneipp therapy, an early form of naturopathy that involved exposure to cold in the comfortless grey hours of early morning. It was named after Sebastian Kneipp, a Bavarian priest, who had purportedly cured himself of tuberculosis largely by immersing himself frequently in cold water. Kneipp—and my mother, his fervent new acolyte—believed firmly that the forces of nature could be harnessed to cure people of disease. Ice cold baths and walking barefoot through dewy grass (or better yet, snow) were essential pillars of his therapeutic philosophy, and a perfect way, as my mother saw it, for two teenage boys to start their day. When she was on a mission it was difficult resist her proselytizing.

Aside from the double shock of being thrown out of bed at dawn and getting our feet thoroughly wet and cold, we felt surprising well. It was true: these odd exercises certainly woke us up and somehow prepared us for the day. In fact, as I would learn many years later, most alternative treatments are pleasant enough. But, like so many other enthusiastic proponents of naturopathy, my mother had allowed herself to become persuaded that Kneipp therapy would also keep us healthy forever, a hypothesis that, I am glad to report, was allowed to go untested: after a few months her enthusiasm for "Kneipping" had thankfully waned and we were able to return to a more lazy normality.

Normality? Perhaps that's not the right word. Our family was anything but normal.

Life in Germany after the devastation of the Second World War was not easy. My father, like his father before him, was a doctor. He had served in Hitler's army as a physician, first on the Western Front and then in Russia. There he became a prisoner-of-war and was lucky to survive the experience. He was a man who loved to tell long stories, but the details of his time as a POW in Siberia remained steadfastly shrouded in silence: not once did he yield to our attempts to learn more about what happened.

Before the war, my parents had lived in Silesia (now Poland). My mother and grandmother had fled the advancing Russian army together with an old family friend whom everyone called "Tante" (aunt), and my two older siblings: my brother (who was not even one year old), and my sister, who was just four.

The little I know about their escape I learned from a memoir that my mother left us. In life she, too, found it hard to speak in any depth about the ordeal, but she did mention that at one stage she was sure my brother would die. What came across most strongly, both in her memoir and in her limited conversations with us about those times, was her absolute determination to stay ahead of the advancing Russian troops who, she felt sure, would have raped the three women and very probably killed the entire group. Together, they had to pull a handcart for hundreds of miles to reach the relative safety of Wiesbaden in the American-occupied zone, which is where my paternal grandparents lived. By then everything of value had been traded or sold in an effort simply to survive.

My father was released from his Russian prisoner-of-war camp about two years after the war had ended, and when my parents were reunited, they must have been so delighted that they produced me.

Like many post-war German families, my family had to struggle for bare survival. I was too little to remember much of this period, but my mother's memoir recounts the incredible hardship as well as the ingenuity these dire times created. There was little coal to heat, nothing to eat and there were no clothes to dress us kids; one of my earliest memories relates to some very scratchy trousers which apparently my mother had made of an old swastika flag she had found somewhere. There was little hope: morale was extremely low and merely the instinct to survive kept us going.

Food was so scarce that my father decided to apply his botanical knowledge from medical school to produce a plant-based powder that, as he confidently asserted, could be used as a flour substitute. Apparently it tasted horrible — so horrible, in fact, that none of us wanted to eat the cake my mother made with it. Meanwhile my grandmother, who was the nicotine addict of the family, took to smoking rose-leaves and parts of the tomato plant; they actually do contain some nicotine, I later found out.

My mother, unwilling to rely on my father's flour-making experiments, would pull the old handcart through the country-side in search of something to feed the family. One day, she came across a heap of onions in an abandoned garden. As she had never been a good cook, the family did not find the taste of the onion soup all that surprising. Two hours later, though, we were all in hospital having our stomachs pumped: she had poisoned us with a soup made out of hyacinth and narcissus bulbs!

My father was keen to secure our survival by starting to work as a physician again. He travelled the region to find a place where he could start afresh. Eventually he found what he had been looking for but it meant relocating the whole family to Bad Neuenahr, a spa town south of Bonn. My father was hopeful that he could re-establish himself there so that we would be protected from starvation or poisoning from my mother's ersatz onion soup.

Before the war, back home in Silesia, my parents had run a little rehabilitation hospital mainly for diabetic patients. My father had been its only doctor and my mother had grown into the role of hospital manager. Now, they had rented a sizable house in Bad Neuenahr where they could put their pre-war experience to good use and start all over again. Soon they were back in business and in charge of a small but well-run institution.

Things were looking up, for there was certainly no shortage of patients. Most men returning from the war were ill. Sadly, that also included my father. His health never truly recovered from his time in Siberia and, on more than one occasion, we saw him at the brink of death. My recollections are vague and hazy but I do remember feeling deeply insecure and frightened being taken to his bedside and saying farewell. Luckily, he lived until his early 80s but we had many tearful goodbyes both assuming it would be the last. A little boy's dream occurred to me: how wonderful it would be to become a doctor and be able to cure him of his various ailments!

The war had destroyed more than just health and houses. Families were breaking up at a record pace — and sadly mine was no exception. In the early 1950s, when I was about 4 years old, my mother and father split up. According to my mother, my father was a serial adulterer; according to my father, it was Hitler's war that had destroyed their marriage. When my parents divorced, the family was torn apart yet again. My mother had to leave all of us three children behind.

Without her, we kids felt lost, sad, abandoned and scared. But there was no choice, and besides, nobody asked us how we felt about this drastic change in our lives. We clung together, became even closer, and tried to carry on as best we could. My father hired a nanny to look after us. We hated her but that changed absolutely nothing, except to unite us even more. Times were hard for everyone, and we were expected to cope and do our best to not make things even harder. This period of our lives was characterized by steely resolve and a refusal to bemoan our fate: navel gazing was stringently discouraged.

My mother had fought hard to start a business in Silesia; after the war, she had to repeat the experience in Bad Neuenahr. Now she embarked on her third, fortunately last and most successful struggle to get settled in life. Virtually penniless, she moved south to Bad Tölz, a spa town in South Bavaria, where she did the only thing she knew well: she rented a sizable house, hired staff on credit and opened a rehabilitation hospital, similar to the ones she had been managing before.

Times were still very hard and, although my grandmother stood by my mother all her life, few others helped her. The exception was my mother's uncle, Hans Jüttner. He seemed to have some money and my mother had the expertise, so the two became business partners. However, when Hans, who had lost his first wife to cancer, remarried, his relationship with my mother quickly soured. My mother ended up by buying him out, and Hans moved away with his new family.

But there was another, less obvious, reason for the split, one we rarely spoke about: Hans Jüttner had been a general in the Waffen SS, an unsavoury pedigree that proved to be a deterrent to prospective patients at the hospital. If nothing else, my mother's decision to separate the still small and fragile business from any Nazi taint was a shrewd move; it saved her reputation, and that of the hospital, and made her the sole owner of what was to become a sizable venture.

We kids were, of course, keenly interested in finding out about Hans' past, not least because any questions about the Nazi era evoked such obvious discomfort in our elders. But, whenever we asked about him, we were told with uncharacteristic conviction that he had been a regular soldier who had done nothing wrong. This assessment was lent greater weight when, during the trial of Adolf Eichmann in Israel, Hans Jüttner gave written evidence for the prosecution, against

Eichmann. Apparently Hans had once disbanded a transport of Hungarian Jews and had later given Eichmann, who was of inferior rank to him, a piece of his mind for instigating such disgraceful activities.

My memory of "Onkel Huscha", as we called him, is that of an elderly, bespectacled gentleman with a quiet voice. His very ordinariness made it almost impossible to imagine that he had once been both a general and a Nazi. This was a paradox that I was never able to resolve satisfactorily. The stubborn irreconcilability of these two personae — the outwardly mild-mannered, lovable Onkel Huscha behind whom lay a history of deep involvement with the Nazi regime — seems in hindsight to embody one of the central mysteries of the Nazi era. How was it possible for millions of ostensibly decent, civilized people to embrace evil with such unquestioning enthusiasm? I have often wondered whether the interest I later developed in researching the history of medicine under the Nazis had its genesis in those early attempts to make sense of the inscrutable past.

***

It took my mother several years of invincible determination to get her children back. Being the oldest of us three, my sister Elga came first. My mother then ran out of patience with my father's stalling and kidnapped my older brother Endrik. She waited until he had been sent to a holiday camp on Germany's north coast, and then secretly drove to the location and simply snatched him off the street. My father protested to no avail. Eventually, at the age of 8, I was allowed to join them. My grandfather had become convinced that I needed to be with my mother and urged his son to send me to her, my brother and sister.

Finally, we were together again. For me, this was a dream come true. We had only been separated for four years or so — but those four years represented half my lifetime, and were certainly long enough for me to have lost almost all recollection of them. I had yearned and begged to be with them but, when we met again, I did not even recognize them.

In the intervening years I had become a peculiar specimen of a boy—shy, introverted and deeply insecure. I did not make friends easily. On the very first day at school in the little Bavarian town where we now lived, I was singled out by my classmates as being unusual and, as a consequence, was beaten up. I had done nothing wrong; I just spoke with an accent that was different from their broad Bavarian dialect. Those Bavarians, I quickly learned, were not exactly overflowing with tolerance.

When I did make friends, it was frequently with the wrong type. With one boy I even experimented with pyromania. It had all started quite innocently with little fires in the woods, but then we somehow got carried away and were caught setting fire to our family home. This was the closest, I think, my mother ever came to hitting me. My poor friend had caught the pyromania bug much more severely than I: he later managed to burn down a couple of houses in town and was sent off to a psychiatric institution to be treated. As fate would have it, his father became my mathematics teacher. Even though this had been my favourite subject, somehow I never achieved good grades during that period.

When it was time for me to go to high school, at the age of 11, I was sent off as a boarder. I had grown close to my sister and brother and both of them had already gone to similar institutions. I had hoped to join them but my track record for unruly behaviour and non-conformity had earned me a place at a different school, one that was famous for its rigour, strict rules and high academic standards. I hated the idea of having to leave home yet again, but despite my protests I was given no choice. I loathed every minute I spent at that school; it felt like prison— which was quite possibly the specific intention of its founders— and to me the teachers, in their unbending zeal for enforcing subordination and total adherence to arcane and often absurd rules of conduct, seemed to be modelled on the guards of a concentration camp.

Determination is a trait I must have inherited from my mother, for soon I became as resolved to return home as she was determined to keep me there. When all my pleading fell on deaf ears, it became clear that only the most dramatic of measures would accomplish the desired aim. I worked hard on my plan and, after only one and a half years, I succeeded in getting myself expelled for unruly behaviour. Yes, I was a peculiar boy, no doubt about it. I did not fit into any of the standard templates, and the efforts of my elders to force me to conform only seemed to redouble my desire to find my own path, no matter how unpopular that might prove.

***

Both my parents' businesses eventually took off during the time of the German *Wirtschaftswunder*[1] in the early 1960s. Most Germans were working hard, very hard—but not us children. None of us ever excelled at school. My sister was the least academic of the three of us; her solution to the problem of escaping the pressures of school as well as the tensions at home was drastic but singularly effective: she got pregnant at the age of 18 and married. My brother, like me, found his teachers uninspiring and his schoolwork dull and pointless, but eventually got his *Abitur*[2] and went on to study law in Munich. As for me, I could not bring myself to take any of this stuff seriously. With few exceptions, my teachers seemed to me to be small-minded failures with an unhealthy zeal for the authority which their position conferred on them. They appeared to view the primary purpose of education as the imposition of constraint, to be facilitated by the frequent administration of discipline and punishment in generous measure. They were at best indifferent to the very principles that are fundamental to education—the instillation of a hunger for knowledge, an appreciation of beauty and art, as well as the encouragement of critical thinking.

---

[1]   The period of rapid economic expansion and prosperity that began after World War II.

[2]   High school graduation exam that serves as a certificate of secondary education.

Indeed many of them treated such notions as downright seditious, a direct challenge to their primacy and to the very system that had set them in authority—a system with which, from the very start, I seemed to be set on a collision course.

I had considerable difficulty accepting authority, and the more I began to think independently, the more I rebelled. Most youngsters are like that, of course, but my insurrection was more than purely a problem of puberty. It had set in well before that period and has persisted throughout my life.

How could it have been otherwise? I have always felt slightly ashamed of being born a German. On several occasions, while travelling abroad and talking to non-Germans about our Nazi past, my shame became acute, almost visceral. Not all of my German friends understood my feelings in this matter; they would argue that the past had nothing to do with us, the children who were born after the war. Pragmatically, perhaps they had a point: it was not us, after all, but our parents who threw rose petals in front of Hitler's motorcade. Nevertheless, it seemed to me that the stain of the past could not be expunged simply by the passage of time. The emergence of a new generation did not, in and of itself, provide absolution. It was our duty and our responsibility to delve into the past, to confront it, ask questions and find answers.

As a boy growing up in post-war Germany, I felt that the actions of my parents' generation were at once unfathomable and unforgivable. As children we watched television, documentary after documentary about the war. When no deeper understanding emerged, even after long and embarrassingly unsatisfactory discussions with the older generation, I felt utterly lost.

At school, we learned next to nothing that, in my view, was meaningful about the Nazi period. Of course, there were history lessons, and we were provided with a sequence of events, particularly those relating to the war itself—but these details appeared somewhat beside the point. The real questions for me lay elsewhere. How could all of this have been allowed to happen? Why did hardly anyone protest? How could I bring the atrocities of this period in line with the notion of a civilized society? This shameful past in which almost all of my elders had been involved in one way or another stripped them of any legitimate basis for directing or criticizing me.

Intuitively, I think, my mother understood why I so regularly and vehemently chafed against authority. She even encouraged protest to some extent and seemed proud that her children were developing into a bunch of non-conformists. To be regarded as "normal" had a pejorative undertone in my family; to be normal meant to be mediocre, dull and average. All of us kids were unusual in some way, and all of us were determined not to repeat the mistakes of the previous generation.

My mother was the most gentle and loving person one can possibly imagine, and there was rarely any reason for conflict or confrontation between us—at least, until her remarriage to "Onkel" Klaus, as we were obliged to call him. Klaus was the coldest fish in the guise of a human whom I had ever encountered. He was regularly the focus of our fiercest and most desperate debates. He was the sort of German who foremost inspired one question in me: What did you do during the war? Entirely unfair perhaps, but the three of us simply could not stand him, and I certainly felt that he had no right to interfere in my life. Not once did he contribute to it in a positive way and far too often he made it an utter misery. This man never made even the slightest effort to understand his stepchildren; on the contrary, he seemed to positively enjoy the often palpable unhappiness and the loaded atmosphere in our home.

Klaus loved to pontificate about how useless our generation was. All we could do, in his opinion, was to criticize and live off the money of those whom we did not even respect. Not once did it occur to him that we were lost and were having a hard time finding our way through the gargantuan mess the previous generation had bequeathed us. He went on and on—and he had it coming; after bottling up my anger for a while, one dinnertime I finally burst out: "Isn't it lucky that we are not as well-organized and efficient as you? Like this, we will never manage the logistics of gassing six million Jews." He went all white and, before he could say a word, I got up and left.

Children as a rule do not find it easy to accept any new partner of their parents after a divorce, and it would have been easy to view my dislike of Klaus as being simply due to jealous resentment of a boy who adores his mother. While I do not claim that I was above such feelings I do not believe the intensity of my dislike can be entirely explained in this way, particularly as I had already been entirely capable of accepting, even loving, my father's new wife.

My father had remarried while I was still living with him, and I certainly had been ready to loathe any outside intrusion into my life at this early and vulnerable stage. But my step-mother Ingeborg turned out to be quite a wonderful person and the absolute opposite of Klaus. She contributed one new child to our family almost every year; in total, she gave me nine half brothers and sisters. As this new family grew, she never once made the slightest distinction between her own children and me. My half-sisters and brothers were lively, to say the least, and consequently my father's house would often give the impression of being a cross between a youth hostel and a lunatic asylum—but it was run by a loving and lovable landlady. In later life, I regularly came to visit them in their huge house. Each time I was struck anew by the overwhelming chaos that reigned there. This realization evoked a strangely dissonant reaction in me. On the one hand, I felt a deep-rooted sense of familiarity and belonging but, on the other hand, I could not help being aware of the profound differences between us.

***

If in my childhood I had butted heads angrily with authority wherever I saw it, as a teenager and young adult this tendency had matured into a somewhat more subtle ability to anticipate and nimbly sidestep the track that others had carefully laid out before me.

By the mid-1970s, my mother had created a fast-growing empire of rehabilitation hospitals. Well, perhaps not quite an empire, but to me it seemed like one, with over 500 resident patients cared for by about 200 staff.

Originally, my mother had trained as a laboratory assistant — which was how she had met my father back in Silesia — and, not being a doctor herself, she employed a team of about 25 physicians to look after the patients, while she performed the roles of general manager, chief executive and planner of the future. As far as she was concerned, my destiny lay in becoming the medical director of this business.

Yet I was in no hurry at all to get into harness and trot obediently towards my predestined future. At the age of 12, I had discovered music in a big way — music in the form of jazz, that is. In the 1960s, most teenagers were buying Beatles records, yet my brother and I were enthusiastically listening to Jelly Roll Morton and Bix Beiderbecke. We loved jazz; it was different, it was fun, and it was music that only a few decades previously had been forbidden in Germany.

My brother and I shared everything, including our passion for jazz; we were best friends. He was the one who taught me about life's mysteries which, at that stage, mostly meant about sex and alcohol. I adored him and looked up to him but, at the same time, I always had the feeling that he was somehow vulnerable: he seemed to need my support, advice and even protection, a phenomenon that has endured all those years to the present.

After both trying our luck on the banjo for a few months, we realized that a two-boy-banjo-band might not be the fastest approach to musical fame. We decided to draw lots; my brother won and opted to keep his banjo, so I switched to clarinet, and later took up drums. Together with some like-minded friends, we formed a small band. We might not have been all that good, but we certainly were enthusiastic and spent most of our time and energy on perfecting our skills.

At the age of 17, I went to school in Seattle. This had been arranged by an American teacher who had visited my school in

Bavaria looking for suitable students to spend a semester at his school in the Pacific Northwest. I volunteered, thinking this would be an exciting adventure. I desperately wanted to get out of the stiflingly smug atmosphere of Bavaria and was eager to put as much distance as possible between Klaus and myself. But, on the morning of my departure, I got distinctly cold feet — colder by far and much more unsettling than anything the early morning Kneipp therapy of my childhood had induced. Some things look so much more attractive at a safe distance: going to live with complete strangers on the other side of the globe suddenly seemed a bit too courageous for my own good.

Nevertheless, I managed to jump over my own shadow and flew all the way to Seattle where, at the airport, I was met by a welcoming committee of students from the White River High School in Buckley, Washington. They were very sweet and some of the girls were good looking — which was a matter of considerable importance to me, as I was hell bent on losing my virginity in the USA. But, to my horror, these lovely people took me to a tiny village in an isolated rural area some 50 miles outside Seattle. I felt even more stranded there than I had in Bavaria. What on earth was I to do in this backwater?

At first, small-town America was fun. I did make friends with some unusual characters, had some real excitement while fishing (illegally) for salmon in the White River; went to school dances, drank beer (illegally), drove a car (also illegally), ate exotic food and wrote long letters — mostly to my brother, whom I missed frightfully.

But just as I had feared, life in Buckley quickly became very boring. The school was so undemanding that, even in English classes, I was the best of my class. To my amazement, I was actually homesick. Foremost, I missed my mother and my brother. And even though I was the only male clarinetist among five females, the daily band classes were no longer doing it for me. In the homeland of jazz, I felt the need to be back home and play jazz with my friends. When it was time to go home, I was more than delighted.

***

In 1966, when I was 18 years old, my brother and I escaped the claustrophobic atmosphere of Bavaria and left for St Tropez. At the time, he was a law student and I was still in high school. During the summer break, we had assembled a small group of fearless musicians consisting of my brother on banjo, two friends from another local band on trombone and drums, and myself on clarinet. We called ourselves The Red Hot Bootleggers—mainly because Jelly Roll Morton's band in the 1920s had been The Red Hot Peppers, but also because by then we had developed a keen interest in distilling—until my mother found out, that is.

Like Jelly Roll Morton, Bix Beiderbecke and so many jazz musicians before us, we now befriended alcohol in no small way; jazz works much better that way, we thought. We won a couple of prizes, a radio contract and even made a record. And it was fun, so much fun! It did not bother us that traditional jazz was an acquired taste, that all the girls went for the boys with the guitars, nor that most barbarian Bavarians had never heard of Jelly Roll or Bix. I loved everything about making music and had little ambition to do much else.

For about four weeks that summer we slept on the beach and, as soon as the afternoon heat was beginning to subside, we installed ourselves in St Tropez's picturesque harbour. Soon we had recruited a fifth man whose sole but crucial task consisted of collecting money from the people who were lounging in sidewalk cafés and on the terraces like sitting ducks. Despite the lack of trumpet and bass, which are normally considered essential for our type of jazz, we were a resounding success, perhaps not musically but certainly financially.

After busking for 2-3 hours, we counted our money—a small fortune by our standards—drank copious amounts of beer and ate voraciously. Later, we were often invited to play on one of the yachts or in one of the posh hotels. At midnight, we would start our only regular job—the resident band in a strip club. That lasted until 3am and could have been a bit dull had it not been for a special treat. We had befriended one of the girls who regularly did a show just for us—a teenager's dream! After a hard day's night, we invariably felt hungry again and would make our way to a little chip shop, the only place open at 3am. The counter girl looked exactly like Brigitte Bardot, or so we thought; the only time we met her while we were sober, her resemblance to the film star had inexplicably vanished.

The way we saw it, our St Tropez excursion had been such a spectacular success that we decided to repeat it the following summer, only this time with a full six-piece band. The music sounded much more impressive now, but paradoxically the excitement was not quite the same. On the journey down, we stopped over in Northern Italy for rehearsals and several extensive wine tastings — perhaps too extensive, with hindsight. The two newcomers in our band first shaved each other's heads, then decided they did not really like each other nor their new mutually inflicted hairstyle, and ended up chasing each other around a parking lot threatening to kill one another. There are some things in life that are so strange and unexpected that any attempt to understand them is doomed to failure.

The determination with which my brother and I were pursuing music by this time must have alarmed our mother. After all, I was destined to become the medical director of the family empire, not to play jazz in dubious clubs for little pay. Endrik was still keeping his head above water at law school, but I had little intention of doing anything other than playing music. My mother knew me well, of course, and must have realized that putting her foot down would have only generated more protest and a determined antipathy to the career path she had chosen for me. So she gently persuaded me that music was fine — not just fine, in fact, it was great, she said — "But why not do both?", she offered. "You could go to the conservatory *and* study medicine at the same time. That way you would have a solid profession to fall back on, if ever you get fed up with making music."

This wasn't a bad plan but there were obstacles. Soon after moving to Munich, I enrolled at the conservatory to study percussion, drums having by then become my favorite instrument. But starting a career in medicine proved to be considerably more difficult. At the time, it was far from easy to enter medical school. Throughout Germany, they admitted only those students with the very best grades—the ones who had sat in the front row, who had studied industriously and who had been the teachers' darlings. I was nowhere to be found amongst this elite. Never having been able to take teachers, learning and that entire scholastic nuisance seriously, my grades had always been less than stellar. This meant I had to join a long queue of frustrated would-be doctors waiting to enter medical school.

To my mother, this was absolutely unacceptable. Like any proud parent, she had always believed that her children were far too exceptional for mundane things like waiting in line; to her mind, we were born in the fast track. Not to be defeated, she came up with an ingenious plan: if she could somehow obtain a testimonial from some suitable source, which expressed in no uncertain terms the notion that, aside from perhaps Albert Schweitzer, the world had never seen a man more destined to become a doctor, the medical school admissions authorities would surely make an exception and instantly throw the doors wide open to the medical school for me. So she sent me to a psychologist who specialized in finding the ideal profession for hesitant adolescents like me. For two days, he made me fill out forms, do exotic tests and answer probing questions. Then he looked sternly at the pile of paper he had amassed and promised that he would analyse the data and send a report, together with his bill, to my mother. We waited with increasing anticipation, and then, at last, it came. His verdict? He felt I was ideally suited to be a crane driver! Needless to say my mother was apoplectic with fury. I am not even sure that the hapless psychologist ever got paid.

Psychologists and psychology, my mother decided, were the pits. But I, for one, was now deeply intrigued. In general, I was rather uncoordinated, had two left hands and was mildly afraid of heights, as anyone who knew me well could have testified. Yet this man had examined me for two full days and had arrived at the bizarre conclusion that my destiny lay in manipu-lating heavy loads from place to place from the dizzy heights of a crane, at considerable risk to those who worked on the ground below. Not easy to get things wrong more profoundly, I thought, and wanted to know more about this bewildering field. So I enrolled to read psychology at the University of Munich.

To be a student in Munich, at a safe yet not too frighteningly long distance of about 40 miles from home, felt liberating and excitingly grown-up. I shared a flat with my brother who was still reading law and seemed to be studying even less hard than I. We had such intense fun that, within weeks, we managed to get evicted from our flat. We were playing in the same band, The Jazz Kids, sometimes five times per week. Music, I was not unhappy to notice, seemed to be winning over medicine after all.

Moreover, the psychology course was rooting itself down in me, and it must have been around this time that a broader interest in pseudoscience began to emerge. At school, my favourite subjects had been maths and physics. Even though I still had only a vague idea of what constituted real science, I was beginning to develop a sense of what a poor imitation of it looked and felt like.

Psychology in the mid-1970s seemed to be an area heavily populated by those who had chosen this subject predominantly as a means of sorting out their own personal problems. We studied Freud, graphology and a weird type of physiology that, as I later discovered, was remarkably different form the real thing. What we would now recognize as post-modern concepts dominated the scene: truth seemed to be relative, and facts elastic. In certain areas of psychology one explanatory narrative was as good as the next, if not better.

This troubled me greatly. After a childhood during which my questions about the country's recent history had so often met with awkward silence and unconvincing rationalizations, I had hoped that psychology might provide a means to arrive at some generalizable, irreducible truths about human behaviour. Instead, I was being offered a steady diet of speculation. Science, I slowly began to understand, provides us with a set of tools that may lead to the truth, if applied correctly. Pseudoscience, by contrast, could only lead deeper into a labyrinth of half-truths.

I had been wandering in this academic wilderness for about a year when my mother's prayers were answered: I was admitted to medical school.

On the one hand, I was delighted: I had come to the end of my patience with psychology and was eager to immerse myself in something slightly more rigorous. On the other hand, I was also a bit apprehensive: somehow I got the feeling that entering medical school was like going through a heavy door that would close behind me with a sombre custodial clang, leaving no possibility of turning back. The days of leisure and contemplation, of laziness and long, boozy nights, were well and truly over.

At this stage of my life, I had been in a relationship for several years. My girlfriend and I had a large circle of friends; we liked to ride—even had our own horses—and went skiing regularly. I was tall, lean, sporty and reasonably attractive. I had enough money to spend, not least through playing the drums in clubs on a regular basis. I was determined to take life easy and not too seriously, if at all possible. I enjoyed concerts, travelling, discussions and perhaps most of all I appreciated anything that made me laugh: when there was a prank to be pulled, I was likely to volunteer. I could find an open bar at 4am and I knew where to listen to the best jazz in town. I was a pacifist, a lefty and an agnostic. I normally disapproved of violence; the only time I ever hit someone was when a local neo-Nazi refused to pay our band. (When I realized that we were not going to get our hard-earned money, I put him flat out—but seconds later, as his bodyguards came after me, I regretted that action.)

How on earth would I be able to continue what I considered "real life" with all this hard work coming up? How would I manage to combine music, hobbies, sports, social life and studies? The answer was simple: something had to give, and it was not going to be medicine. Deep down, I knew that only too well: my life was indeed about to change in a very fundamental way.

When I look back with the benefit of hindsight, I cannot help viewing my younger self rather disapprovingly as something of a dilettante, a spoiled brat. It's true that I was privileged in many ways, and I did not always behave responsibly. But the intervening years have erased much of that devil-may-care attitude, and age has conferred a generous measure of cynicism and perhaps even a little wisdom. Even so, the blueprint for the person I would eventually become was very much present and discernible in the young man I was then. I am still unapologetically iconoclastic and mischievous. I still love music, laughter and wine. As for psychology, I still love the idea of magic — we all do — but I have grown exceedingly wary of pseudoscience. However compelling and beautiful they may be, illusions are still lies. And when it comes to embracing lies — and acting on them, sometimes with murderous zeal — humankind has a lousy track record.

***

Getting to grips with the seemingly endless flood of medical knowledge was hard — even harder than I had anticipated. The curriculum was packed and, crucially, at the start of medical school, it was also bone-dry and often seemingly irrelevant and mind-numbingly boring. We were being turned into little robots with no time to think for ourselves, and no time to question what was demanded of us. I had wanted facts and now I found myself learning millions of them — well, perhaps not millions, but it certainly felt like that.

My fellow students in the psychology department may have been a trifle neurotic and self-absorbed but many were nonetheless quite original, fun-loving personalities. My medical colleagues, by contrast, seemed more like learning zombies trying to conform eagerly to everything they were told. For me this was infinitely disturbing: I had grown up habitually objecting to authority and doubting most things that were presented to me as facts. Yet medicine seemed full of dogmas which were just crying out to be challenged—but there was never the time to analyse and question them critically.

I was determined not to become like all the other medical students around me who seemed to live just from exam to exam. Yet, I had to concede that they had a point: we had little choice but to be conformist, obedient, hard-working robot-like creatures hectically mopping up knowledge, simply because there was such an overwhelming amount to be absorbed.

In truth, non-compliance with the schedule would have been deeply irresponsible not just because of the consequences of failing the next looming exam but also because, one day, it might lead directly to harming patients. Almost all the facts we had to learn were important, particularly in the second phase of our studies when subjects like biochemistry, physics or zoology had been left behind and we were trying to understand the complexities of the human body and mind. For a physician, lacking a sound knowledge of basic facts might one day mean the difference between the life and death of one of his patients!

At school, I had often felt that we were learning for the teacher—which was why I mostly refused to comply. As a psychology student, I had the impression that many of my fellow students were studying with very personal motives. As medical students, we were learning for the benefit of our future patients—and the medical school faculty made sure that we understood that immutable fact loud and clear.

I had my share of frightening experiences that brought home this message forcefully. In my second year, I worked in a small country hospital during the summer vacation. I remember being asked to administer intravenous injections to all the patients of one particular geriatric ward. The matron had pre-pared a tray full of syringes and gave me detailed instructions as to how the task was to be completed. "You start in the first room and make your way through the entire ward. Every patient gets a different injection. They are already prepared and ordered in sequence." German doctors are great believers in injections, as are their patients: when medication is injected there is no possibility of overlooking a dose or forgetting to take a pill or of malabsorption due to illness, etc. My supervisors had, of course, taught me how to safely insert a needle into a vein and had made quite sure that I mastered this task reliably. I was proud of having acquired my first clinical skill, but the prospect of injecting real patients with real drugs made me tremble and sweat. There was no way to chicken out, so off I went and administered injection after injection — there must have been at least a dozen — gaining confidence as I went. All seemed to be going fine until, about one hour into the job, I had almost finished my round and was attending my last patient, and the matron caught me. "What are you doing still with the first patient?" "Not the first", I replied. "This is the last." When we realized what had happened, we both rushed through the ward to check how my patients had taken it. Instead of doing my round clockwise, I had done it anti-clockwise. Every patient, except the one right in the middle of the sequence had therefore received the wrong injection. Miraculously, they were all fine. Not just fine, they seemed very pleased with my service. Sooner or later all physicians realize that most patients are resilient enough to withstand most of their errors. Thanks to those hardy geriatric patients, I had learnt this important lesson well before graduation.

***

Doctors on the whole aren't well known for understanding and sympathizing with their patients' emotional needs. When it comes to appreciating the vulnerabilities of patient-hood, there is no more useful or instructive teaching experience than for a doctor in training to become a patient him- or herself.

In my case, that opportunity came when I was involved as a passenger in a head-on car collision. It happened during a visit to London; two friends and I had decided to visit my old friend Philip who lived there. Philip and I had met years ago in France, where we had both gone to learn French but, of course, once we became close friends Philip learned no French and I learned nothing but English during that summer.

There we were in suburban London, returning from a good evening out. It was 3am. I was riding in the back seat, singing loudly. Philip, the only sober person in the car, was driving when another car, driving on the wrong side of the road, hit us at great speed.

The full extent of my injuries was only discovered when, after two days in Epsom hospital, I was flown back to Germany. Up to this point, I had been walking about, albeit with difficulty, but now I was told to lie flat on my back and not to leave the bed—not even for the "essentials". I had broken my lumbar spine in two places and there was a real risk of becoming paralysed.

The medical team decided that it would be best for me to spend a total of three months in bed—and that's exactly what I did, never once leaving it. To depend in this way on the help, expertise, good will, generosity and kindness of others was an overwhelming experience. Even though I was rarely in much pain, I was frequently desperate. Every visitor told me how lucky I had been, and obviously this was true and I knew it. But, at the same time, there's only so much stiffness one's upper lip can bear before it begins to curl into an angry rictus. The prospect of three months staring at the ceiling, of having to go through a lengthy rehabilitation process afterwards, of being isolated from everything I loved, of having chronic back pain for life, or worse—perhaps even losing sexual function—was dire and depressing. The fact that I had so much time for brooding made keeping depression at bay infinitely more difficult. There were moments when I wished Philip had driven a bit faster and it had all come to an end there and then. I had always seen myself as a cheerful person, yet during those three months in bed I got to know a new and much darker side of myself—one that was not so easy to live with and one that I never wanted to meet again.

The experience gave me more than enough time to view my future profession from a different perspective. It made me realize just how important factors such as compassion, kindness, empathy, understanding, dedication and time really are.

For the very first time, I grasped with clarity and personal immediacy the concept that patients are not just "cases" but vulnerable individuals. The experience showed me dimensions of medicine which I had hardly noticed before. Of course, as a patient I wanted the best, most advanced, most effective therapies. But I also needed human warmth, sympathy and loving care.

As a medical student, I had heard all of this in lectures and had read about it in books, naturally. But theory only takes us to a certain point. To experience incapacity and injury from the patient's perspective brought the truism home to me: medicine is indeed just as much an art as it is a science.

Patients, I now know, tend to put more weight on the art of medicine—even just the caring bedside manner—than most health care professionals realize. Without it, patients often experience medicine as dehumanizing and traumatic. Physicians, on the other hand, tend to focus on the science of medicine. They often overlook the human side of patient care, mostly because they have, or pretend to have, too little time for the compassion and empathy that are so central to the art of medicine. Instead, they tend to delegate this important function to the nursing staff. But being a good doctor requires that both the science *and* the art of healing be brought to the bedside. Medicine that omits one of these essential elements is incomplete: it may be health care, but it's not good medicine.

As it turned out, I was supremely lucky and, despite the two spinal fractures, I made a full recovery. Apart from occasional back pain, I suffered no lasting consequences of the car accident. None of the other passengers had been severely injured either. Three months in bed had even provided me with ample occasion for the much-needed catching up with my preparations for my final exams at medical school.

In the late 1970s, "finals" consisted of a long series of face-to-face interviews—about 30 in total—stretched out over almost half a year. We were asked to form groups of four students, to stick together throughout the entire ordeal. The four of us used to meet at increasingly frequent intervals, and I realized that the other three were just as scared and just as unsure of themselves as I was. The schedule was so tight that we often only had one or two days to prepare for the final touches in what we termed "minor subjects", such as ears, nose and throat (ENT).

We had learnt basic ENT during our studies, and then we had revised it with all the other subjects at the outset of our final preparations. Now, as the exam approached, we had given ourselves little more than one day to refresh our memory. On the big ENT day, we were ordered to arrive at 7am at the professor's office, an unholy time by anyone's standards. The building was still locked, so we rang the bell and waited; eventually a blue-collar worker, whom we took to be a janitor, opened the door and asked us to take a seat in the professor's waiting room. Ten minutes later, the same man arrived dressed all in white and announced: "As none of you recognized me opening the door to let you in, I assume that you were not the keenest attendees of my course. So let's see how well you are prepared."

As far as I was concerned, his judgment was spot on. Since I never had any intention of earning my living looking into other people's orifices, I did not consider ENT a priority and had decided to give his lectures a miss. Now, it seemed, I was about to pay for my sins.

After this disastrous start to the exam, things only got worse. Our tormentor thought it would be fun to have the four of us examine each other, and one of my fellow students was thus ordered to examine and describe the state of my tonsils. Before I could say a word, she had nervously rammed her spatula down my throat and started fantasizing. If her actions had not so effectively silenced me, I would have been able to warn her that my tonsils were not "slightly enlarged and mildly inflamed", as she began describing them. In fact, they were totally absent; I had had them out at the age of 12. After glancing into my throat himself, the professor triumphantly exclaimed: "He had a tonsillectomy many years ago, you fool." At this stage, my poor colleague's nerves cracked and she started crying. I looked at everyone in turn and reacted as I often do when under maximum pressure: I had a laughing fit.

This tendency to burst into uncontrollable laughter at moments of unbearable tension had got me into trouble before when I was a boy at school. No good trying to suppress it, that only made things worse. I remember one of my school reports had even mentioned: "Prone to disruptive laughing fits." My teachers had always interpreted this habit as disrespect, but luckily our ENT professor did not draw the same conclusion; in fact, he joined in and, within seconds, all five of us were crying with laughter and unable to stop for several minutes. When we finally did sober up, the professor seemed to have changed his mind about us. He started asking some reasonable ENT questions and, as luck would have it, we even gave a few sensible answers. In the end, we all passed.

Not that all of our examiners were so kind and forgiving. By far the worst was our neurology exam where the professor was patronizing, condescending, ill-tempered and arrogant from the start. Neurology, it turned out, was yet another subject that was not exactly our forte. We had prepared diligently, but somehow this man had an uncanny knack of searching out the most embarrassing gaps in our knowledge. Once he had identified a weakness, he would dwell on it punitively — and most inelegantly, I felt. Yet, even to him, it must have been clear that we had worked hard and that we knew most of what he wanted to know. When finally it was all over, he passed us but, on leaving, he put on a smug smile and said: "Send me a postcard when you open your own practice, so that I can avoid ever becoming your patient."

By that time, this six-month-long exam marathon was almost over, which was just as well: our nerves were wearing thin. The two girls were crying too often; my male colleague confessed that he was not sleeping or eating normally, and I was drinking too much. Our very last exam was "Functional Anatomy". Our knowledge of basic anatomy had already been tested years before during the pre-clinical period of our studies and, to me, even that had been something of a nightmare. No other subject in medicine is so overloaded with ponderous terminology and minute detail. Functional anatomy had the potential to be even worse, for it required the ability to relate the physical features of anatomical structures to their physiological function. In the anatomy exam they might, for instance, have asked what muscle is supplied by which artery and by which nerve and is attached on which bone or tendon. In the functional anatomy exam, they could ask you to explain what these facts meant in the context of the function of the limb, and what would happen if any of the elements in this hugely complex muscle, tendon, bone, artery, nerve-unit were injured or went wrong—not my favourite subject by any stretch of the imagination, I have to admit.

This time, our examiner was a middle-aged female professor. She too had ordered us to her offices at 7am. She knew that this was our very last exam. Amazingly, she apologized for the ungodly hour, explained why she was unable to offer another time, gave us coffee and biscuits and started chatting. How had it gone so far? What were our professional plans? What were our hobbies? She seemed intrigued to hear about my enthusiasm for jazz and was convinced that she had heard me play somewhere. Finally, after about 40 minutes of relaxed banter, she proceeded to sign the paperwork. That was normally the sign for the exam to be concluded. I looked puzzled. "Something wrong?", she asked with a smile. "I thought you would examine us." "If you insist! Follow me." We went next door where she had prepared part of a cadaver for the examination. She took a scalpel and pointed at the nose. "What's this?", she asked. "I'd say it's a nose", I said, and frantically tried to remember the nerve and blood supply of this organ as well as all the conditions that might cause the sense of smell to become impaired. "What's the function?" "To smell", I answered. "Quite right, you have passed."

Chapter 2

A Doctor at Last

After six seemingly never-ending years of medical school, I had finally qualified as a doctor at the not so tender age of 30. On the way home, I stopped my car and had a good cry, a cry of joy and relief. It felt like a new horizon had suddenly opened up. Beyond it lay a future full of uncertainty, adventures and challenges. It was at once terrifying and elating.

Sure, there was much to be proud of; after all, I was now a doctor! But how would I cope with the pressures of the job? What if I turned out to be a dismal failure? Like most junior doctors, I was profoundly insecure about my abilities. Was I mature enough to be a good physician? So far, I had gained the impression that most people found me likable enough, but was this true or was I deluding myself? As much as I doubted others, I doubted myself even more.

The celebrations were long and wild, but even the most exuberant Bacchanalia must eventually come to an end. It was time to find a job. What on earth did I want to do with the rest of my life?

I had managed to navigate through school without ever working hard or taking it seriously. I had fallen in and out of love several times. I now was in a steady relationship but was nevertheless strangely unfulfilled. I had gone through medical school without serious problems. Thus I had proved to myself and the rest of the world that I was able to work hard and achieve things, if I had set my mind on them. My future as medical director of the family business had been mapped out for me since I was a child at my mother's knee—yet I felt little enthusiasm for rushing into that career. I was not an indecisive person by any means, but now I had to confess that I was more than a little uncertain where I was going.

So far, I had been atypically hesitant about becoming a physician. Yes, I did want to follow in my father's and grand-father's footsteps, but it had never been an irresistible urge; and neither had I ever seen myself as a likely candidate to pursue an academic career. The decision to go into medicine had been difficult mainly because, first and foremost, I longed to be a musician. The moments of my life in which I had experienced intense happiness and weightless joy had occurred not during my years as a doctor in training but when I was on stage behind my drum-kit, playing together with inspired musicians. What would have been ideal was a life that combined both music and medicine, but these are both jealous lovers and neither could have been easily persuaded to move over and make room for the other. As it was, I felt torn between the two: the clinician in me was just taking his first diffident steps; the scientist had not even awoken, and although I was now undeniably a full-fledged physician — with a freshly-minted diploma to prove it — I still felt much more like a musician than a doctor.

To complicate things further, finding a junior doctor's post in the late 1970s was far from easy. Germany had a surplus of physicians and the most attractive hospital jobs seemed to all be taken. With the help of our family doctor, I eventually found a position in a place that, at the time, was Germany's only homeo-pathic hospital. Our family doctor had been a good friend of my mother for many years and, after hearing about my predica-ment, had phoned his colleague, the hospital's director, who had promptly offered me this post.

Moving into homeopathy straight after medical school might have been an odd choice, yet it seemed fairly unremark-able to me. Our kind family doctor, who, like many of his German colleagues, often used homeopathic remedies along-side standard medicine, had treated me in this way since child-hood. The impression I had formed through this early personal experience was that homeopathy was often effective. Most

German physicians would use homeopathy with the vague idea that it somehow helped the body to heal itself. They would employ homeopathic remedies mostly for non-life-threatening, chronic diseases, particularly those for which conventional medicine had no cure (for example eczema, allergies, hay fever, sleeplessness, irritable bowel syndrome or headache). For more serious diseases, they would invariably turn to the standard armamentarium of conventional drugs.

As a young boy, I once fell acutely ill with colic of some kind. The pain was excruciating. Our doctor was called and treated it successfully by injecting a mainstream drug. Another time, I had caught a mild form of infectious hepatitis. He monitored my liver function and gave me homeopathic remedies. My liver subsequently normalized, and we all concluded that homeopathy had worked. I am sure this sounds utterly bizarre or even irresponsible to most modern physicians but, to me, it seemed entirely normal.

The relatively peaceful coexistence of homeopathy and conventional medicine in Germany is bewildering to people who have not grown up with this duality. How can doctors claim they are grounded in science and, at the same time, tolerate or even practise a type of medicine that is as remote from science as astrology is from astronomy? I am not sure that I know the answer to this question even now, and back then I had not yet started wondering.

As it was, my theoretical knowledge about homeopathy was close to zero. At medical school, homeopathy had rarely been mentioned but I had, of course, heard from our professor of pharmacology that this type of medicine was complete and utter nonsense. Pharmacologists tend to become particularly enraged when anyone mentions the "H-word" because homeopathy contradicts almost every single principle they teach.

Since I was about to start my job in the homeopathic hospital, I quickly read up about homeopathy. What I learnt was more than bewildering. In a nutshell, homeopathy is based on two main assumptions that were described by Samuel Hahnemann about 200 years ago. The first is often called the "like cures like" principle (*similia similibus curantur*, in Latin). Hahnemann asserted that, if a substance causes a certain symptom in a healthy person, it could be useful in treating these particular symptoms when they occur in a patient. This might sound elaborate or complicated but, in fact, it turns out to be surprisingly simple: because my eyes start watering when I am chopping onions, for example, onion is a homeopathic remedy for treating hay fever—which is, of course, characterized by watering eyes.

The second principle is often referred to as the "memory of water". To use the above example of the onion as a remedy for hay fever, homeopaths do not use the pure onion extract. Instead they dilute and shake, and dilute and shake the extract many times over. They call this dilution process "potentiation" to indicate their conviction that it renders the remedy not less but more potent. Dilutions are often in steps 1:100, which is characterized by the letter C (*centum* is the Latin for one hundred). A typical homeopathic remedy is so watered down that it no longer contains a single molecule of the original substance. A 'C30' potency of onion, for instance, would contain 1 part onion extract in 1,000,000,000,000,000,000,000,000,000,000,000,000,000,000,000,000,000,000,000,000,000 parts of water. Another way to express this is perhaps even more explicit: for a "C30" pill to contain just one single molecule of the substance printed on the label, the pill would have to have a diameter similar to the distance between the earth and the sun. Once we have fathomed this simple premise, we can immediately see why scientists find homeopathy so hard to swallow.

Homeopaths acknowledge the fact that the repeated dilutions may indeed result in not one molecule of the original active ingredient remaining, but crucially they also claim that the repeated shaking—a process they call "sucussion"—transfers some sort of indefinable energy from the onion to the water —hence, the phrase "memory of water".

When I began working as a physician in the homeopathic hospital I knew, of course, that homeopathy lacked scientific plausibility. There is no reason to assume that evoking similar symptoms will cure a disease and there is even less basis to the notion that diluting a substance will render it more powerful. But I was prepared to shrug my shoulders and concede pragmatically that if it helps, it helps. After all, I had benefitted from these strange remedies myself on numerous occasions. Perhaps my appointment as a junior doctor in a homeopathic hospital would enable me to get to the bottom of this paradox: on the one hand, homeopathic remedies could not possibly work; on the other hand, they clearly did help some patients to get better. This was an intriguing contradiction, and from that perspective alone the offer of working as a homeopath was a chance I didn't want to pass up. As things turned out, the decision did indeed prove fateful; few of the many posts I took during my early career would turn out to have nearly such a profound and long-lasting influence on my professional life as this one.

***

The Munich homeopathic hospital was housed in a modern building set in a pleasant park in the southern suburbs not far from where my girlfriend and I lived. With only around 100 beds, it was a small but famous and respected institution. The hospital itself was extremely well-run; it was immaculately clean, there was an unusually tight discipline about everything, and the food was the best I ever ate in any hospital anywhere in the world.

In the entrance hall there was a big sign, "Here we do not smoke!", which was not at all typical of hospitals at that time. In the 1970s, smoking was still allowed everywhere, even in hospitals and even on the wards. So the non-smoking policy was way ahead of its time. The wording of the sign was, however, unusual and somewhat patronizing, I thought. It did not simply say "No smoking" or "Please abstain from smoking", but delivered its message in an Olympian tone, almost as a value judgment.

Everyone working in this place was very kind but, at the same time, my colleagues were often pushy, given to minding other people's business and quite unashamedly on an evangelical mission whose goal was to convert everyone to the gospel of Samuel Hahnemann.

Being a "real doctor" was terrifically exciting—at times even more fascinating, I slowly began to feel, than being a musician. Initially, I was merely shadowing more experienced colleagues, but after a few weeks I was given more responsibility. What I saw was impressive. We were treating mostly chronic conditions, anything from asthma to rheumatoid arthritis and from migraine to obesity—lots of obesity. Despite the fact that we were dishing out remedies which, as my pharmacology professor had insisted, contained precisely nothing, patients usually did get better, some even dramatically so. I was bowled over! Soon I found myself treating my mother, siblings and friends for this or that minor illness. Even our dogs did not escape my enthusiasm for the newly discovered pilules containing sugar and… sugar.

Yes, I was impressed, but occasionally I also had doubts: was it really the remedy itself that was responsible for the recovery of our patients, or was it the careful, compassionate attention paid to the patients that brought about their improvement? Perhaps the patient would have improved even without any therapy at all? Crucially, was not every young doctor impressed when treating his first patients and watching them recover? Was I perhaps deluding myself about the powers of the ultra-diluted homeopathic remedies? These nagging doubts stimulated reflection and made me eager to explore further and learn more.

The medical director was frequently a tad tyrannical with his staff but he seemed to like me and took me under his wing. So we frequently had long discussions about all sorts of issues. His reply to my question "What precisely causes the improvement of our patients?" amazed me with its disarming honesty. "It's mostly due to the fact that we discontinue all the useless medications they had been taking previously." I had not previously thought of that possibility at all.

But it was true: we did scrap most of the unnecessary drugs. I was struck by the amount of nonsensical prescriptions many patients had accumulated during the often long years of their medical history. All these drugs did, of course, have the potential to cause side effects. Throwing them overboard was therefore quite likely to improve our patients' symptoms, provided these drugs were truly superfluous. All this was hardly amazing and even my pharmacology professor would surely have approved. What was remarkable, however, was that my boss did not claim that his miniature homeopathic pellets were the prime reason for the improvement. Perhaps he did not himself believe in homeopathy? Such heretical thoughts!

The placebo effect, I suggested, might be another reason for homeopathy's success. During my time in this hospital, I witnessed many instances of its amazing power. Once, during a ward-round, a patient experienced an acute asthma attack just as we were passing by her bedside. I had never seen anything like it; within minutes she seemed to suffocate in front of our very eyes. She was deteriorating fast into what I thought was a critical state. I was alarmed, if not panicked. My boss, however, remained strangely calm: "Don't worry," he told the patient, "we will give you an injection immediately. It will have an instant effect. Trust me; you will be fine in just a minute." With that we all left the room; outside, the nurse was instructed to prepare a saline injection. This, we all knew, would have no effect at all; saline injections are pure placebos. I was told to go back to the patient and administer the injection intravenously. I was horrified: how could this help a patient on the brink of death? But when I argued my corner, my concerns were dismissed peremptorily.

So I did my best. On arrival at the patient's bedside, I continued reassuring her that my injection was powerful and would be dramatically effective. And to my utter amazement, so it proved to be. Seconds after I had injected the saline, the patient began to breathe regularly, her colour normalized, and she relaxed.

"Never forget the incredible power of placebo", my boss later told me. He was absolutely right, and I never did forget the importance of placebos. In fact, years later they actually became a focus of my research.

That first hospital job in Munich also taught me to practise a range of other alternative therapies besides homeopathy. I was usually taught new techniques by doing them, the expectation being that I would read up about the subject in my own time. A famous saying put it in a nutshell: watch one, do one, teach one. During my time at medical school, I had already attended courses in acupuncture and what was known as autogenic training, a method of self-hypnosis that teaches patients how to relax effectively. Now I learned elements of herbal medicine, of cupping, neural therapy, treatment with leeches and other exotic therapies.

One of my colleagues even practised dowsing, a bizarre diagnostic method. Whenever he was not sure which homeo-pathic remedy to prescribe, he would take out his pendulum and brood over that patient's case notes until the swing of his instrument told him which the right treatment was. Even in the eccentric atmosphere of the homeopathic hospital, this was considered to be fringe medicine. We used to smile at this pro-cedure and had our doubts about its validity. But nobody ever challenged him, or asked him to explain exactly how the swing of his pendulum could reliably resolve a thorny clinical or therapeutic dilemma. It was instances of this kind that, after a few months, began to kindle in me an increasingly urgent need to move on.

It had already occurred to me that some of my colleagues used homeopathy and other alternative approaches because they could not quite cope with the often exceedingly high demands of conventional medicine. It is almost understandable that, if a physician was having trouble comprehending the multifactorial causes and mechanisms of disease and illness, or for one reason or another could not master the equally complex process of reaching a diagnosis or finding an effective therapy, it might be tempting instead to employ notions such as dowsing, homeopathy or acupuncture, whose theoretical basis, unsullied by the inconvenient absolutes of science, was immeasurably more easy to grasp.

Some of my colleagues in the homeopathic hospital were clearly not cut out to be "real" doctors. Even a very junior doctor like me could not help noticing this somewhat embarrassing fact. One particular physician, for instance, made an extraordinary fuss each time she had to give an intravenous injection. Her inability to do this properly often resulted in pain, bruising and distress for the patient, generating a complaint — and this, of course, made her even more nervous and flustered the next time she was called upon to perform the procedure. Each injection thus became a major event disrupting the entire ward. In the interests of protecting the patients as well as preserving an atmosphere of peace on the ward, I decided to do the injections discreetly myself, before she even had time to panic. Once she had discovered that this task gave me no problems, she regularly delegated all the injections to me. Who knows whether she ever learnt to master that simple and essential technique?

One day, we were to perform a liver biopsy on a patient. This was a very big event in the off-beat environment of the homeopathic hospital, way outside our comfort zone. The task fell, of course, to the most experienced doctor, whom I volunteered to assist. Already during the preparations, he seemed exceedingly nervous. When he finally pushed the horrifyingly thick, long biopsy needle through the patient's skin in the direction of her liver, he turned white and then promptly fainted. The patient was in considerable discomfort, and I was left attending to both of them. Eventually I attracted help and we managed to pull out the biopsy needle and obtain what looked like a decent tissue sample. The biopsied tissue was then sent off for analysis. Two days later, the report arrived on our desk. The first sentence was very disrespectful of our endeavours. "Thank you for sending us this '*schaschlik*' (the German word for a mixed meat skewer one might order in a restaurant) for histological analysis." It turned out that we had sampled bits of our patient's diaphragm, lung and liver.

Fortunately the patient was blissfully unaware of any of these problems; she had not experienced any suspicious symptoms and survived our incompetence quite splendidly.

***

I left the homeopathic hospital after about six months. Subsequently, I worked in several conventional hospitals in the areas ranging from general medicine to surgery and rehabilitation medicine. Eventually, I secured a post at the University of Munich in the Department of Rehabilitation Medicine where I was expected to engage in all three elements of university-based medicine: patient care, teaching and research.

I had never anticipated or planned an academic career but, when they offered me this post, I thought why not? It certainly fitted perfectly with my mother's master plan of me becoming medical director of the family business, and she was delighted. In fact, both my parents were very happy: my mother saw things going very much as she had hoped for the family concern, and my father was pleased that at least one of his many children would follow him into the medical profession.

Most junior doctors have to work long hours and nights and, by then, I had done my fair share of that too. Now, my clinical work mainly consisted of looking after patients in a busy out-patient clinic. This meant marvelously regular working hours, starting at 8am and usually ending around 6pm. Best of all, there were no night or weekend duties. This gave me enough time for making music and for pursuing other interests. At this stage, alternative medicine had become somewhat of a hobby. I enjoyed hands-on training in massage techniques and spinal manipulation, and occasionally I also practised the alternative therapies with which I had already become familiar. Again, I was lucky: I had a very kind boss who soon became a close personal friend.

This was a peaceful, happy time for me, and an important period in my professional life. I found my feet, gained valuable experience as a clinician and became much more focused in terms of narrowing down a direction in which I hoped to develop. This was the time when I became a real doctor, able to differentiate between the important and the unimportant in patient care, capable of listening attentively to patients, confident in my abilities and able to cope with clinical routine as well as with the unusual events and crises that medicine always has in store.

During this period there was a surprise of quite a different kind in store for me also. Dramatically and unexpectedly, totally and uncompromisingly, I fell in love.

I was playing with The Jazz Kids at a gig in London. Danielle, a French woman aged 25, then living in London, came to the club where we were performing. At first, she assumed that I was a musician by profession. We talked, danced and were instantly attracted to each other. It quickly became more serious; attraction turned into passion and passion turned into love. I was entirely overwhelmed. To complicate matters, we were both already in relationships.

For a short while, we managed to keep our love secret. We both needed a little time to reflect. Were we really sure about all this? Perhaps it was just an infatuation? No, it certainly wasn't. Neither of us had ever felt like this before; nothing else seemed to matter any longer and no obstacle could have stopped us. I simply adored her — and still do. We just had to be together.

The hardest thing was to tell our respective partners: neither of us wanted to cause pain. In comparison, the rest seemed almost easy: I gave notice at my job, informed my totally surprised mother, brother and sister, packed up a few things, drove to London (stopping at my father's house on the way), rented a flat in Chelsea, and started a new life with Danielle.

Chapter 3

A Golden Cage

An entirely new phase of my life had started. Now that Danielle and I were together, it seemed as though I could achieve anything I wanted; I felt adventurous, strong, happy and reborn.

Initially we rented a tiny flat in central London and were having such a wonderful time that I hardly noticed that I was not working. But we were living off our savings and, after about three months of this idyll, our funds were nearly exhausted and we were forced to move to the suburbs.

I needed a job. I had been confident that I could easily work anywhere: surely in a big city like London it would be easy to find employment—but I couldn't have been more wrong. As had been the case in Germany, there was a surplus of junior physicians during the late 1970s in the UK. I sent off about 500 applications before I was finally offered an appointment—in a psychiatric hospital. Psychiatry was not a field I had ever given much consideration to but, under the circumstances, I felt I had little choice but to accept.

The psychiatric hospital was housed in a huge, gloomy Victorian brick building just outside London. Although I had no psychiatric training or experience, I was immediately put in charge of more than 100 in-patients on what were euphemistically called "long-stay" wards. In addition, I also had to look after an acute admission ward and do all sorts of other things, some of which I found deeply disturbing. Every Wednesday afternoon, for example, it fell to me to administer electroshock therapy to patients suffering from severe depression. To say that I found this duty distressing is an understatement. The patients were terrified. They felt, I am sure, like the victims of inquisitorial torture, and most of them submitted to this procedure only against their utmost physical resistance. They had to be strapped down and gagged before the treatment could take place. The memory of those gruesome sessions has haunted me ever since. To me, psychiatry felt like medicine from the dark ages: cruel, punitive and, above all, based not on science but on speculation and supposition.

The longer I worked in this place, the more I hated it. Night duties, in particular, were not just unpleasant but positively scary. By far the worst aspect was that I did not feel that my work was helping anyone. When I visited the wards, the nurses usually wanted me to increase the dose of sedatives of patients who had been "difficult" the night before. I remember a case of an elderly lady: because her diagnosis was unclear to me, I insisted on seeing her complete case-notes which amounted to half a room full of files. She had been a patient of this hospital for decades. Once I had fought my way through this mountain of paperwork, I realized that this poor patient had never been adequately diagnosed as being clinically ill. On the contrary, I got the impression that she had been admitted because her family felt she was nuisance. Naturally, she protested, which led to her being branded by her nurses as "difficult". As far as they were concerned, my task now was to keep her from being "difficult" by sedating her up to the eyeballs. Since she had long since developed adverse effects from the drugs, I refused to comply on medical grounds. Subsequently, I was told that my refusal was counter-productive and cruel, as they would now have to physically restrain her.

The last straw came when I found out that several of my female patients were in the habit of prostituting themselves at night to passing truck drivers outside the hospital walls. When I tried to stop this monstrosity, I was told to mind my own business and to not "rock the boat" — after all, the wretched women badly needed the pocket money.

After almost six months in this hellhole of a hospital, I left. Since then, rocking the boat has become a familiar occupation. Boat-rocking has the potential to initiate real and rapid progress —but it is also a sure way of making powerful enemies.

***

Homeopathy, psychiatry—where next? Until now I seemed to have made my way in medicine by a process of exclusion, stumbling rather haphazardly from one unlikely position to another, serially discovering my aversions rather than purposefully pursuing my preferences. But then, as luck would have it, I managed to secure a post in a research laboratory at St George's Hospital in London, for which I did indeed have some qualifications even though my recent experience as a failed psychiatrist cannot have been much of a recommendation.

The research group hiring me was a world leader in the field of blood rheology, the study of the fluidity of blood. The group was investigating why uncoagulated blood, under certain circumstances, behaved almost like a solid, while normally it is quite fluid. The research involved measuring the viscosity of blood and its constituents under defined conditions and developing methods to quantify the deformability of blood cells.

My previous experience of the scientific method had been during my final years in medical school, back in Munich. During this time, I had decided to write and present an M.D. thesis. (This is a necessary precondition in Germany for being permitted to use the title "doctor".) My thesis concerned blood-clotting abnormalities in women experiencing septic abortions, a very dangerous situation where an infection, often from an abortion gone seriously wrong, spreads rapidly throughout the body. This research had certainly taught me a lot more than the average doctor learns about blood clotting and the complex phenomena involved in this process. It had also taught me something about research techniques, the skills of laboratory work and the basic principles of statistical analysis.

Now these skills had to be hurriedly resurrected. In 1979, the clinical departments of St George's hospital had not yet moved from Hyde Park to Tooting in South London, and the new St George's Hospital, where I was, was still under construction. This meant that we had plenty of time for long discussions with the few members of staff who had already been relocated to the new site.

I quickly became totally absorbed in the work we were doing. I felt that our research was of fundamental importance and that the phenomena we studied had immediate clinical relevance. For example, we studied the deformability of red blood cells. The human heart pumps blood through arteries that become narrower and narrower as they take the blood to tissues further away from the heart. Eventually the diameter of these tiny vessels becomes even smaller than that of a single red cell. If blood cells were not extraordinarily deformable, they would not be able to squeeze through these tiny tubes and the circulation of blood would be impossible. As these cells deform in the tiniest capillaries, they come into very close contact with the surrounding tissue. This is how vital processes such as the transfer of oxygen and other substances from the blood cells to the tissues take place. Any condition that limits blood cell deformability, I began to realize, is potentially precarious. Finding treatments that could restore the flexibility of red blood cells might thus be useful for a wide range of conditions.

All this was very exciting, not least because, for the first time in my life, I found myself amongst scientists and a whole group of very bright people. We travelled to conferences, gave lectures, published papers, criticized our own and other scientists' work, and planned new research projects improving on previous studies. Medical school, understandably, had been almost exclusively clinically focused; it had done very little to hone my skills as a researcher, critical thinker or scientist. Now that I became immersed in the world of basic and applied research, I was beginning to realize how vital the scientific aspect of medicine really was.

Another wonderful aspect of my first serious encounter with science was that I was given plenty of time to think, read, learn, discuss and write. Almost every day, for example, I spent time in the library—a great luxury that those who practise clinical medicine are seldom granted. Clinicians hardly ever have enough time; the next patient is usually already waiting. My boss was a case in point: he was first and foremost a surgeon, and his clinical duties meant that he spent long hours in theatre, leaving me very much in charge of managing my own time and investigations. The free and relaxed atmosphere of the research lab gave the team ample opportunity to debate the results of the most recent experiments and to plan the next round of studies. We frequently hosted visitors from abroad and regularly consulted colleagues who worked on related projects. This open and, to me, characteristically British exchange of ideas taught me more than any textbook ever had. For the first time in my professional career, I felt I had found my vocation: I was able to take a step backwards and look critically at my previous years as a doctor.

Clinicians are far too often the victims of the circumstances they have to work in. We treat our patients the best we can in the hope they get better. If they do, we are, of course, delighted and almost automatically conclude that our treatment has been successful. In other words, we assume cause and effect mostly because the postulated cause (i.e. the treatment) preceded the effect (i.e. our patients' improvement). Hardly ever do we have the time, sense, inclination or humility to doubt this rather simplistic notion, and hardly ever do we question or criticize anyone for making it.

In a way, our most fundamental assumption in clinical medicine is like suggesting that the first crow of the rooster before dawn is the cause for the sun rising. In order to establish cause and effect, one must take into account many more factors than simply the correct time sequence. Receiving a treatment today and getting better tomorrow might suggest that the treatment caused the clinical effect, but it certainly does not prove it. Such seditious thoughts were entirely new to me: it was exhilarating to analyse and to begin thinking scientifically in this way.

Scientists try to control the circumstances of their experiments in such a way that cause and effect can be more clearly determined. They are systematically taught to doubt and criticize even their very own concepts and results, because this helps them in designing better and more conclusive experiments for the future. An uncritical scientist is a contradiction in terms: if you meet one, chances are that you have encountered a charlatan. By contrast, a critical clinician is a true rarity, in my experience. If you meet one, chances are that you have found a good and responsible doctor.

I spent roughly two years at St George's, planning, conducting and publishing rheological experiments. It was the steepest learning curve and the happiest time of my life; I did not even miss making music all that much. Luckily my boss, even though notoriously short of time, was a wise and kind man. I owe him a lot: we became, and still are, good friends.

But much though I loved the work, the atmosphere of the lab and the company of so many intellectually stimulating colleagues, I was beginning to feel the need for more clinical experience. After all, that's what I had studied medicine for: I wanted to be able to apply the theoretical insights from the laboratory to the treatment of patients who were suffering from vascular diseases. In addition, of course, there was always the nagging background awareness of the family business, and my mother's serene expectation that, one day, I would cease my restless questing and come home to take up the position for which she felt I had always been destined. But I just wasn't ready for that yet, and when a hospital near Munich offered me a post with a view to combining my research in blood rheology with clinical work involving patients with severe circulatory problems, it seemed like an elegant solution, and I accepted.

When I left St George's I took with me a corpus of knowledge and expertise that enabled me to continue research in the same area. More importantly, I took with me the capacity to think analytically, critically and scientifically — and, as it turned out, this ability would determine the rest of my professional career. Perhaps even more crucially, I took with me an abiding love and appreciation for Britain that eventually drew me back to the UK and, in 2000, impelled me to embrace British citizenship.

***

The typical patient who came into my care in my new position would be a middle-aged male smoker with critical leg ischemia that was threatening the survival of his legs. We would try to improve the blood flow such that an amputation could be averted. This was often far from easy: the major arteries supplying the legs can be irreversibly blocked and, at that point, the best approach usually is vascular surgery. Sadly, surgery is sometimes not possible or not successful. In such cases, the only other option is to improve the fluidity of the blood to restore the blood flow in tiny vessels that are capable of bypassing a blocked artery.

The scientific expertise that I had acquired in London seemed to fit perfectly into this clinical context. My new boss was visibly impressed with the list of research papers I had managed to publish during my time at St George's and hoped that he and his unit might benefit from the continuation of this work. Few things in medicine, I began to understand, are more important than a long list of publications. Many doors open more easily if one has been regularly published in *The Lancet* or similar journals of high standing.

Ostensibly, I had been employed as a scientist with some added clinical duties, and I had hoped to divide my time about half and half between these two tasks. Yet the reality turned out to be very different: for the first six months not the slightest attempt was made by my superiors to let me do any research at all. I never even had as much as an hour to set up the expensive equipment that had been bought but had never been put to use. Worse, I began to suspect that my boss would not recognize good science even if he fell over it. It soon became clear to me that I had been misled: nobody in this institution was truly interested in science. They only wanted research, or even just the appearance of being research-active, as an enhancement to their reputation, but certainly not for enlightenment. My time was taken up looking after seriously ill patients, attending needlessly long ward rounds and writing or correcting long, tediously detailed doctor's discharge letters.

German hospital medicine has always been obsessed with these documents. In theory, they are supposed to inform a patient's GP in a timely way what diagnoses and treatments have been established during the patient's stay in hospital, so that care can be continued smoothly once the patient has been discharged. These letters have always been the bane of junior doctors everywhere. They are first drafted and then corrected, and then re-corrected *ad nauseam*, often by nit-picking senior colleagues who rejoice in the opportunity to demonstrate to the juniors how superior they are. Finally they are mailed, often far too late to be of any use to anyone. Every hospital and every consultant insists on their very own style to which junior doctors have to adapt each time they change post.

The aim of these needlessly wordy documents, it seemed to me, was not so much to be helpful to the patient and the GP but more as part of some archaic ritual aimed at humiliating juniors. German medicine must be the most formalistic and autocratic healthcare system in the world. Many rules, regulations and customs exist not because they are useful but merely because they have always existed.

After working in England, the "German way" came as a rude awakening to me. In London, it had been accepted that the juniors were on a learning curve. It was expected and encouraged that they ask questions rather than covering up gaps in their experience and knowledge. Equally, British senior colleagues were never too embarrassed to ask younger colleagues about something they had once learnt but long since forgotten. In Germany, by contrast, everybody had to pretend to know everything; uncertainty or doubts were interpreted as a telltale sign of weakness. Questions were perceived as indications of incompetence rather than eagerness to learn. The structure was rigidly hierarchical, with the juniors at the bottom, and by general consensus this was where they belonged. The boss could—and frequently did—get away with all kinds of nonsense; he was a semi-god who was not to be doubted, questioned or criticized. At the other end of the scale, the junior doctors were expected to be hard working, devoted, obedient, servile and uncritical of their superiors. The patient, who should have been at the centre of all this activity, did not really matter all that much. Sometimes it even seemed as though patients were deliberately used to demonstrate the superiority of those at the top of the pecking order.

Needless to say, this atmosphere rubbed me up very much the wrong way. It ran counter to most of my newly acquired insights about critical thinking and open discussion of different views or options. It was a hindrance to obtaining valuable experience or making progress. Experience became synonymous with the ability to repeat mistakes over and over again, instead of learning from them. Inevitably, I began getting into conflicts with my superiors, and it didn't take long for me to realize that this hospital was a place where neither science nor health care could thrive. As a consequence, I expressed my views openly and resigned.

Throughout my professional life, I have been extremely fortunate to be able to take this sort of risk without undue hesitation or circumspection. Whenever I quit a job, I had the full backing and support of my family and friends. Later, when I had to fight much more important battles, the moral support of family and friends turned out to be crucial. Some people think that I am, on occasion, foolishly courageous in standing up for what I think is right. This compliment—and I do see it as a compliment—is, however, only partly justified because I always had the necessary support and security that enabled me to be able to follow my moral compass.

As it turned out, I had loyal friends indeed. My former boss from the Munich university department of rehabilitation medicine picked up the pieces and offered me a post to rejoin his team. He had never been Teutonically dogmatic, a national characteristic that I had come to loathe. The reason for his open-mindedness was simple: he was not German; he came from Hungary, a country where I was soon to make many more friends.

But despite this generous and kind offer, I hesitated; my situation was complex. The vacancy was not for a scientist, but unambiguously for a clinician. As much as I wanted to accept, I was determined—now more than ever—to continue my research. The solution to this dilemma was found when my friend managed to change the job description for me: I was offered what looked like the ideal job—mostly research with some modest attachments to clinical routine and teaching medical students—an offer far too good to refuse.

The job started auspiciously: after a few months, I had managed to obtain grant money to buy the essential instruments and, a little while later, I was able to offer a job to a colleague who had become my successor in the London lab. He too was Hungarian and, originally, he had been one of the many visitors to the St George's team. He arrived in Munich with his wife and two little daughters who all seemed to be pleased to be closer to home.

Soon we were running two labs in parallel, one in Munich and the other just outside Munich in one of my mother's rehabilitation hospitals. We were conducting exciting and well-funded research. Our results were of sufficient interest to be published in some of the best medical journals. They were internationally recognized, so much so that I was able to write, submit and pass my PhD without difficulties. In addition, I founded my first medical journal, *Perfusion*, which still exists today.

Amazingly, I had managed to import something of the London scientific spirit into the unlikely environment of Bavaria. We now had an innovative research unit, and we were more productive than we had ever been before. At the core of our research were two sizable population studies for which we had measured the fluidity of the blood of two very large groups of people. Subsequently we had shown that these measurements predicted some clinical outcomes of those individuals in their later life. This was intriguing, and we were convinced that we were on to something important.

Meanwhile, Danielle and I had been living together for some years. I proposed marriage on the occasion of a visit to Wiesbaden, my birthplace. Back in Munich, I enquired about the necessary formalities. This confirmed the impression I had gained previously: the Germans are the undisputed world champions of bureaucracy. The officials insisted on an extravagant amount of paperwork and formalities. Some of the originals were in French, so they wanted translations, rubber-stamped by a notary. "And what, if we flew to America and got married there?", I asked. "It's a possibility, but, it's not the same", I was told. Indeed, it's not, I thought, and quickly bought two tickets for Miami.

In the US, we merely needed negative syphilis tests and two witnesses. The former was unproblematic but the latter turned out to be a little more complicated. On our wedding day, we went into a Miami police station where the local sheriff did not take long to understand our predicament. He unlocked two cells and quickly recruited two inmates to act as our witnesses. Before we knew it, we were married and celebrated the event by getting a Coke from a vending machine outside the police station.

***

Medical writing represented a means of bridging the divide between purely clinical medicine and the rarefied world of academic research and this activity became more important to me during this period. During my years in London, I had forged a link with *Münchner Medizinische Wochenschrift*, one of the most prestigious weekly medical journals in Germany and also one of the oldest medical journals in the world. Back then, I had regularly contributed short comments on all sorts of subjects, particularly those related to UK health care. I enjoyed this, and besides, it provided a little extra money. After I had returned to Munich, this journalistic work increased.

Occasionally, the editor sent me to medical conferences and, in 1983, I published my first book with them. Its title was *Klinische Hämorheologie* (Clinical Haemorheology), and I think it sold about 5 copies, 4 of which must have been bought by my mother.

MMW was also the journal in which, in 1981, my first article on alternative medicine had been published. Naturopathy had always been a popular and accepted part of German health culture, and it occurred to me that it might be interesting to use my newly acquired investigatory skills to test this homespun wisdom. With the help of a group of medical students who wanted to complete a research project for their M.D. thesis—just as I had had to do a decade earlier—I set out to examine the influence of a number of different naturopathic nostrums, including regular garlic consumption, on blood rheology. The results were remarkable, and several papers were published. As naturopathy was not an area known for the buoyancy of its scientific research, enthusiasts in this field were excited by our work.

It so happened that an annual scientific award had been set up in honour of Father Sebastian Kneipp, to encourage scientific investigation of naturopathic methods. As this award was highly regarded within the field of naturopathy (and even came with a tidy sum of prize money) I submitted our research—and to my great delight, it won.

Even though I have received over a dozen prestigious awards during my career, I have always had a special affection for the Kneipp Preis. The large framed document still decorates the wall in my office as I write these lines, and when I look at it I am always reminded of my childhood and those early hours when, at my mother's dogged insistence, my brother and I dragged ourselves out of bed in order to shuffle sleepily, clad only in our underwear, through the cold, wet grass.

On a more sombre note, it was also through my association with *MMW* that I became interested in discovering more about the deep involvement of the German medical profession in some of the worst atrocities of the Third Reich. To my horror, I had discovered that *MMW*—"my" journal—had been more than an innocent bystander: some of the experiments performed on concentration camp prisoners had first been reported in its pages. Forty years after these horrible events, it was time to come to terms with our own past, and one way of starting this process was to write about it, I naïvely felt.

However, this turned out to be much more controversial than I had anticipated. Some elements within German medicine —and Bavarian medicine in particular—seemed still unwilling to acknowledge the profession's shameful past. After some unpleasant exchanges, I decided to sever my connection with the journal.

Some years later, I had a rapprochement with *MMW*. After my exit from *MMW*, I had started writing for another locally based medical journal and, as it happened, the two journals merged into one publication. Subsequently I was invited to become a member of the new editorial board. By then I had developed a pleasant, fruitful and uncomplicated relationship with the magazine despite my continuing research interest in the crucial role played by the medical profession in enacting Hitler's murderous racial hygiene policies.

***

Whenever things go really well I tend to get slightly worried: will it last?

My Hungarian friend and co-worker was the brightest and best-educated scientist I have ever had the pleasure of working with. As an ex-Olympic swimmer for Hungary, he was also a picture of a man. I had always assumed that he was destined for great things. His long-term plan was to go back to Hungary when the time was right. Back home, he would doubtlessly have had an impressive academic career ahead of him. Today, all of his Hungarian colleagues with whom we collaborated during the early 1980s are heading university departments. I expected him to do at least as well. But fate had a different plan in store.

We were attending a conference in Vancouver and one evening I noticed that he was not quite himself. Jet lag, I thought. But back in Germany, he still did not perk up, and I urged him to have his blood tested. His leukocyte count turned out to be highly abnormal—no small irony for someone conducting research into blood cells. Further tests revealed he had leukemia—and not a benign form, but a fast-progressing, deadly one.

Initially he had several intensive courses of chemotherapy. Despite the powerful drugs, his energy, enthusiasm and optimism remained unbroken. We conducted dozens of research meetings by his bedside and our work progressed much as before. We were full of hope but the bad news came when he was told the chemotherapy had not totally eradicated the malignant cells in his bone marrow. His only chance to survive the disease was a bone marrow transplant, which at that time was still was an experimental and hugely expensive treatment.

His sister, who turned out to be a close match, came from Hungary to donate her bone marrow, and the transplant was carried out in Munich. To this day, I find it hard to talk about the months that followed. His fight was nothing short of heroic. He survived the transplant but the rejection-reaction eventually killed him. It was a slow and cruel death. I will never forget visiting him in hospital. He was kept in sterile conditions under a tent of transparent plastic and pressed his hand on the cover to touch mine. Modern medicine can be intensely cruel.

He left a wife and two lovely children. They went back to Hungary to bury him in his hometown, Pecs. Several years ago, his friends established an annual scientific award in his name: The Arpad Matrai Award. In 1998 they honoured me with it. So many years later, and still I had to struggle against tears to deliver the memorial lecture.

When all this happened, I was shaken to the very core and, for a while, found myself no longer able to think straight. We all tend to say "life must go on"—and it does, of course. Yet some losses cut so deep that life does not continue in the same way.

Eventually, I pulled myself together and began to reassess the situation. I had lost a dear friend and the best colleague I would ever have. Things were changing at the university, too: the head of department had just retired and his successor was not my cup of tea, to put it mildly. The conclusion seemed inescapable: I needed a change, preferably a dramatic one. I still had no strong sense of where I was bound professionally, but I knew beyond doubt that I needed to move away from Munich and look for a new horizon.

By that time, I had become a certified specialist in rehabilitation medicine. This enabled me to apply for a post as a Professor in Rehabilitation Medicine at the Medical School of Hannover and, days before my 40th birthday, I was appointed. My mother felt as vindicated as she did proud: surely now I would be firmly on track to take up my preordained post as medical director of the family business.

Danielle and I enjoyed Hannover. Although neither the town nor its surroundings were as beautiful as Munich and the mountains south of it, we both found the people of Hannover much more agreeable and open-minded than the Bavarians. The medical school was one of Germany's newest, most modern institutions of its type. My professorial colleagues had a reputation for innovation. Better yet, a spirit of openness prevailed which had never been the case in Munich. Hannover was closer to England, not just geographically but also in spirit.

Living with a foreigner in Munich had been quite an eye-opener. I had almost forgotten how provincial, blinkered and unwelcoming the Bavarians can be. Years back, I had lived in a very rural environment south of Munich. My house was in the middle of nowhere and, as is true of any remote agricultural area, one inevitably relied on help from the surrounding farmers. But, although I had lived in the region for about 20 years, I was still viewed as an outsider by my Bavarian neighbours. It was only after I had stitched up the hand of a farmer's son following a bad injury—I was working in surgery at the time—that some degree of friendliness and cooperation commenced.

The way some Bavarians treat foreigners seems to be dictated by their fabled stubborn pride — at least, they refer to it as pride — but to me, returning from England with a French wife, it often seemed much more akin to naked xenophobia. In Hannover, by contrast, we experienced none of this. Our move felt like a relief and a new start.

My duties at the medical school were mainly clinical. The hospital ran a busy out-patient clinic and also provided rehabilitation for over 1000 in-patients of the large University Hospital. My new boss was a perfect gentleman and could not have been kinder. Unfortunately, though, the clinical demands of the post were overwhelming, and opportunities for re-establishing my research programme were slim. I had grown adept at recognizing the signs of my own impending restlessness: even though I liked Hannover very much and was generally much happier there than I had been during the last months in Munich, I knew that the inability to do research would sooner or later poison the well for me.

It so happened that just then the chair in Rehabilitation Medicine at the Vienna Medical School became vacant. The post looked like an interesting challenge: the new professor was to take charge of a team of about 20 co-workers, move the team into a new, 2000-bed hospital, and expand the existing team into one of 120 staff within the next four years. The result would be the largest department of its kind in Europe. There was no question; I had to apply.

They had invited all four of the short-listed candidates — myself among them — to attend on the same day for the selection procedure. Each university selects its professors differently. In Vienna, the process involved a morning of public lectures by the candidates, followed by a panel consisting of 12 Viennese professors interviewing each of us separately. Nobody likes to be exposed to such an ordeal. Being by nature rather a shy person and not a natural public speaker, I was more than a little apprehensive about the whole thing, and extremely glad that Danielle had volunteered to come along for moral support.

Our flight was due to leave Hannover mid-afternoon but we were packed and ready hours before. As we were killing time in order to avoid being too early at the airport, Danielle had suddenly become flustered: "Quick, we have to go!" It turned out that we had made a mistake; the plane was leaving two hours earlier than we had assumed and we were, in fact, already running late. So we jumped into our car and drove to the airport. Rush hour got us badly stuck in traffic; nothing was moving. When we finally got under way again, our old Volvo started fuming and would not run faster than 20 miles per hour. As we arrived at the airport, we simply dumped the ailing car in front of the departure hall and ran to the desk. "The flight has just left", the ground staff told us. We must have looked so very desperate that they took pity. One of the airline's employees picked up the phone; eventually she was put through to the captain of the plane, which had already left the stand and was taxiing to take off. Amazingly, he, too, took pity on us and asked us to walk out onto the tarmac and approach his plane. He wanted to check how much luggage we had. It was a very small plane, just a dozen seats or so. His fear therefore was that, if he took on more weight, he would have to re-do the trimming. Luckily we only had hand luggage. A minute later, the steps of the plane descended and, right there in the centre of the windswept runway, we were allowed to board.

After that cliff-hanger of a start, I knew that the rest of this journey would be a piece of cake. Nothing could possibly stress me now. The next day, I gave my lecture about the research I had done, discussed my findings with the audience and sat in front of the interview panel to answer their questions. I have no recollection at all of what they asked, nor of my answers, but the interview must have gone well because, later that afternoon, they unanimously voted to offer me the job.

It took a while to sink in. This appointment exceeded my wildest dreams. How did I find myself here — me, the self-confessed amateur medic and would-be professional musician with no ambitions in academia? All I ever wanted was a happy and reasonably peaceful life, preferably punctuated at regular intervals by gigs and musical adventures of one sort or another. At school, I had somehow managed to wriggle through without much hard work. I had studied seriously to cope with the demands of medical school and graduated—but certainly not brilliantly. Then I had drifted from one junior doctor's job to another until, quite by chance, I had caught the science-bug. That certainly had been a turning point: it had made a difference in terms of what I was able to achieve and in the way I looked at health care and life in general.

Ironically, without ever having truly yearned to make a high-profile academic career, I had found myself appointed to be head of an internationally prominent department at a highly respected institution. The Medical School in Vienna had a long and remarkable history. The medical faculty had been established in 1365 and, later, during the reign of Maria Theresa, it achieved worldwide recognition. The General Hospital, which was to be my place of work, had opened in 1784. Famous professors at the Faculty included people like Rokitansky, Semmelweis, Billroth, Lorenz, Freud and Landsteiner. Within the last 100 years, 15 Nobel Prizes had been awarded to professors of the University of Vienna.

Realizing all this, I was more than a little afraid of my own courage. There was a part of me that felt that there had been some mistake: was it really me who they had chosen and not someone with the same name? The professional success of the last decade had given me some confidence, but could I truly master the enormous tasks ahead of me? I was not at all sure of that.

The good news of my appointment came just in time for my mother. I phoned her straight away; she was elated. She had been in poor health for several months, but regardless of all her problems, she took the next flight to visit us in Hannover.

Only weeks later, she had to have heart surgery and never regained consciousness. After 28 days in intensive care she died. I have no words to describe my grief.

***

The university administrators in Vienna insisted that the terms and conditions of my contract be negotiated in minute detail. I can never be bothered with such things and was ready to just sign on the dotted line. Yet they wanted complete clarity and piles of paper needed filling, rubber-stamping and signing. I remember being surprised by the generosity of some of the terms. When it came to my salary, everyone said that this was hardly of any real importance. One well-meaning professor at the medical school explained: "It has no true relevance because you will earn several times your salary on the Golden Mile."

The Golden Mile? I did not know this term. It turned out to be the nickname for the streets surrounding the medical school where virtually all the full professors (called *Ordinarius* in Austria) looked after their private patients in luxuriously equipped private hospitals. So I was going to be stinking rich?

The next thing that baffled me was that I had to become an Austrian citizen. Only Austrians were allowed to become full professors at an Austrian university. This bluntly xenophobic rule had apparently been established after the war to prevent the University falling into the hands of the Germans yet again. Relations between the two countries had not always been entirely amicable. Amongst other things, the Austrians resented the Germans for invading their country in 1938, and the Germans never forgave them for producing the monster that made them do it. But now almost all new professorial appointments were awarded to Germans rather than native-born Austrians. It is typical of Austria, I soon found out, to first create rules and then work out elaborate mechanisms to circumvent them.

When, finally, all the negotiations had been concluded and all the papers had been stamped, signed and counter-signed, I became an Austrian and subsequently was able to get on with the tasks that lay before me. Danielle had found a magnificent house on the outskirts of Vienna. My new team at the medical school seemed friendly and welcoming. Everybody was unfailingly nice—with hindsight, perhaps suspiciously nice. I had brought with me two co-workers from my time in Munich.

Their task would be to help me introduce some much-needed science to my new unit. They too were received warmly. Everything seemed to be going very well indeed.

My most important initial remit was to prepare the move of my department into a brand new building, the New General Hospital. Amazingly, plans to create this institution dated back to the time before the First World War. From the start, corruption had been rife: I was told that one entire local government, many individual politicians and administrators as well as untold millions in funds had vanished in the shadow of enormous scandals surrounding the new building. Now I understood why, on the road approaching Vienna, someone had posted a large sign: "The Balkans start here." I should have taken more heed of that, but, in truth, when I took up my post none of the tumultuous past of the New General Hospital really concerned me; I was just impatient to get on with the task in hand. Besides, what could be problematic about moving into a brand new hospital that was almost finished?

I was about to find out.

My department had been chosen to become the very first clinical unit to populate this new mega-hospital with more than 2000 beds. The next eighteen months taught me how naïve I had been to expect simply to move in and get to work. Right from the start many of the key organizational features of this institution were already hopelessly outdated. The cardinal principle in Vienna seemed to be: "Why do anything simply, if it can possibly be done in a complicated fashion?"

Virtually every other day I sat through exhaustive planning meetings with experts in areas I had previously not even known existed. Initially, I didn't mind this activity; if nothing else, it provided me with plenty new things to learn. But as I got acquainted with the Viennese ways of solving problems, I started to wonder. Corruption seemed to be everywhere and nowhere; I could never quite put my finger on it. This might have been because I had never previously been aware of it and had never truly looked for it; after all, I was a doctor, not a detective.

If, by chance, there was an issue that did not present a problem, you could bet your last shirt that, before long, someone would come out of the woodwork and create one. Complications, it seemed, were an industry in and of itself, not least because they presented rich opportunities for intrigue and corruption. Slowly, I began to realize that many of these time-consuming discussions were just a façade. Whatever there was to be decided had usually already been decided long before. The meetings were skilfully engineered and mainly served the purpose of confirming and rubber-stamping the decisions taken to suit someone else.

The new premises of my department were in excess of 3,000m². One of the hundreds of "decisions" that had to be debated, discussed, re-debated and re-discussed was the colour of the walls. I learnt that there are experts who advise you even on such seemingly trivial matters. Some were experts only in charging lots of money, but neither money nor common sense ever seemed to matter. We were told which colours might have what effects on patients and staff. All very interesting, I thought, but let's just hope the result is aesthetically pleasing. Someone mentioned orange. Certainly not orange, I thought; imagine 3,000m² all in bright orange! It's enough to give us all a headache and turn my workforce into aggressive monsters. Yet, sure enough, for some unimaginable reason this was the colour we got—never mind my protests.

Realizing the futility of these endless pseudo-discussions and sham-meetings, my enthusiasm for hospital planning diminished every bit as quickly as it had emerged. But somehow, all this tedious work had to be done, and eventually we managed to conclude it. On the plus side, I had become something of an expert in hospital design and organization. On the minus side, I had lost one and a half years of my life learning a prodigious number of things that I would never need again.

Finally, we were ready to move into Europe's largest hospital where we would one day provide a rehabilitation service for more than 2000 in-patients, plus run a whole string of busy out-patient clinics.

The opening of the first clinical department in the New General Hospital was considered something of a milestone in the history of Austria—hardly surprising in view of the almost 100 year-long planning history, the political scandals and the millions that had disappeared without trace. There were speeches from politicians and administrators, and there were photo opportunities, videos, interviews, newspaper and magazine articles—every conceivable kind of publicity.

Weeks before the opening I had started wondering what I might say on this auspicious occasion. Because of the medical school's proud and venerable tradition, I considered looking into the recent past of my own department with a view to using a historical perspective for my address. This turned out to be a very bad idea.

The history stopped very abruptly in 1938 when the head of rehabilitation medicine had mysteriously vanished from the official records. Whenever I asked questions about this, I was told, cryptically: "These things are better left alone." "What things?" "You know—1938 and all that." Of course, how could I forget? This was the year of the *Anschluss,* when Hitler's troops had marched into Austria and forcibly unified it with Germany.

Whenever someone tells me to leave an intriguing subject untouched, I am bound to do the exact opposite, particularly if this advice is accompanied by a certain, somewhat threatening, look. So I began to research deeper and deeper into the Nazi past of my department and the Viennese Medical School. This task took much longer than anticipated—years rather than weeks. Consequently, my opening speech was blissfully devoid of historical allusions and entirely uncontroversial.

Most of the relevant documents from 1938–1945 had disappeared. Many people would repeat the initial warning (or was it a threat?) not to research this area: "Some things are best left alone", they would whisper conspiratorially in my ear. Each time I heard this phrase, my interest became more acute and my research efforts intensified. What I found would depress me and make my life in Vienna more difficult than it was already gradually becoming. Eventually it would significantly contribute to my decision to leave.

Despite the fact that I am not trained in a historian's research methods, I felt impelled to finish this research to the best of my ability. Finally, I summarized my findings in an article that was published in the *Annals of Internal Medicine* in 1994. If someone asked me today what might be the most important paper that I have ever published, I would name this one without hesitation. Here is an extract that captures what happened to the medical faculty in Vienna in 1938.

> After 11 March 1938, the date on which Hitler's troops marched into Austria and the *Anschluss* (the integration of Austria into Nazi Germany) was completed, the most drastic changes took place at an unprecedented speed. Almost immediately, 153 of the 197 members of the Faculty were sacked... The dean of the Faculty was replaced on 15 March with an outspoken Nazi, Professor Eduard Pernkopf. Later that month, Pernkopf sent a letter to all University staff: "To clarify whether you are of Aryan or non-Aryan descent you are asked to bring your parents' and grandparents' birth certificates to the dean's office no later than the end of April. Married individuals must also bring the documents of their wives". All professors had to give an oath of loyalty to Hitler, and by 24 March the minister responsible for the University of Vienna had ordered the Faculty to be "cleansed" of Jews and other unwanted persons. On 6 April, the "venia legendi" (license to teach at university) was withdrawn from all "suspects" and, at the beginning of May 1938, Pernkopf submitted to his superiors a list of those of his colleagues who had been unable to take the oath to Hitler.
>
> Little opposition was voiced by colleagues remaining in the Faculty; the whole action was carried out without major disturbances and was obviously both well planned and enthusiastically supported...
>
> ...sterilization had already been superseded by euthanasia, which was done mostly in psychiatric institutions; one of the several infamous... sites was the University's pediatric hospital, where many children were killed. A key person in the killings

was Dr. Hans Bertha; he was awarded a professorship from the Faculty in 1945, shortly before the end of the war…

Other atrocities directly related to the Faculty were experiments done on human prisoners at Dachau; these experiments were led by Viennese professors Wilhelm Beigelböck and Hans Eppinger. Under Eppinger's directorship, Beigelböck was engaged in a project to find out how long humans could survive on seawater. The experiments entailed the torture of many Jews in Dachau. Both professors were discussed during the Nuremberg Trials: Beigelböck was sentenced and Eppinger committed suicide. Pernkopf worked on the publication of an anatomic atlas, which contained material from children killed in a Viennese hospital. His Institute of Anatomy also used the corpses of executed persons for teaching purposes; part of this material is believed to be still in use at the University…

After the end of the war, a law condemning the former Nazi physicians was anticipated but never materialized. It was estimated that the law would have affected most Austrian physicians, which might be the obvious reason for its non-appearance. Of the 200 teaching staff of the Faculty, only 19 were thought not to be burdened by a Nazi past…

At no point did Austrian officials invite back those physicians who had been thrown out in 1938. On the contrary, the new president of the Austrian Medical Association, Dr. Alexander Harwich, wrote to key addresses in London and New York discouraging the emigrants from returning. He reasoned that there were "no Jews left to treat," that there was "a shortage of housing and work," and that the Nazi physicians were "unlikely to leave their posts." Thus, in 1955, only 6 former members of the Faculty had returned. The Österreichishe Ärztezeitung, official organ of the Austrian Medical Association, published a 2-page paper in 1988 to commemorate the 50th anniversary of the events of 1938. They stated that "…of the many University teachers exiled from their home country, only few felt the desire to come back to Vienna following the collapse of the Nazi regime…"

My paper was not published until 1995, by which time I was no longer at the University of Vienna but had left Austria and gone joyfully back to the UK to take up my post at the University of Exeter. When the paper was published it had a considerable impact and important consequences. On the one hand, I received a torrent of hate-mail and threats, and was even accused by the more sensationalistic elements of the Austrian press of having stolen considerable amounts of money from my department at the University of Vienna—an entirely fabricated story, of course, and so ridiculous that I couldn't even take it seriously enough to instigate legal action.

But, on the other hand, the paper led to a lively worldwide debate, some of which focused on the *Pernkopf Atlas*, at that time a much-praised standard textbook of anatomy. When it became clear that its original drawings incorporated the Nazi insignia and might even feature dissections of executed victims of Nazi terror, many experts argued that, despite its undoubted artistic and scientific qualities, it should no longer be used. As a result, most libraries across the globe banned it from their shelves.

But, for the time being, all was still well in Vienna. I was busy getting the department organized and hoped to start a new programme of research. The latter turned out to be much more difficult than it should have been. There was enough money, space and manpower to get on with it but absolutely nothing in Viennese academic politics has ever been that straightforward. Most decisions had to be taken by committees, and all university committees had to be composed of one third non-academics, one third junior academics and one third full professors. Because most professors have a plethora of commitments that frequently take them abroad, they were usually under-represented at these meetings. Consequently, decisions were often unwise and shortsighted and usually went against the interests of this most experienced group of experts.

The most lasting and least agreeable memories of my four years in Vienna relate to the uncounted petty but, at times, vicious intrigues that formed the foundational and most extravagantly time-consuming part of academic life at the medical school. The Viennese medical profession had elevated the skill of plotting against one another to something of an art form. Bizarrely, they were even proud of their intrigues as though they were creations of rare beauty, choreographies of diplomacy and politesse rather than exercises in falsification, extortion and back-stabbing.

As my department was expanding very rapidly—we were recruiting a new member of staff almost every other week—I was particularly vulnerable and constantly on the receiving end of these little plots. Some were disarmingly simple—for instance, a colleague might phone me and suggest that the next vacancy to be filled in my department should go to the daughter, son or cousin of an old friend of his. I would naïvely answer that we would always go through a process of short-listing and interviewing and that the best applicant should get the job. "That is absolutely fine, but if the best person is not my friend's daughter (son, cousin) I will have to make sure that all the 67 outstanding vacancies for your department will be scrapped", would be the typical reply. By citing the exact figure of posts in the pipeline or some other confidential details, that person would demonstrate that he was very well-informed and connected; his threats were therefore to be taken seriously.

Such petty blackmail was an almost weekly occurrence, and needless to say I found it intensely annoying. I remember when it happened to me for the first time, I was so furious that I told my staff I felt like punching the culprit to relieve the tension. They were so impressed with my reaction that they bought me a punching ball to hang in my office. During the years that followed, I used it regularly to decrease my stress level, but sadly it did not solve the underlying problem of the uninter-rupted stream of intrigues that came my way, stole my time and made my life difficult.

The stereotypical Viennese solution to being cornered in this way would have been to instigate a counter-intrigue. For instance, you could consider teaming up with another colleague who owed you a favour from a previous plot. With a bit of luck, he or a friend of his could dish some dirt on the original blackmailer. Subsequently you could let him know, preferably through another middleman, that you had something on him. Finally a deal could be struck whereby the blackmailer abandoned his quest and you would forget about whatever you had learnt about him.

Such "tit for tat" behaviour was going on constantly. I tried my best to stay out of it where I could but, sadly, this was not always possible. As time went on, I inevitably got drawn more and more into this ugly morass. Apart from finding the constant intrigues and counter-intrigues distasteful, primitive and degrading, these activities tended to drag you deeper and deeper into the mud, thus rendering you more and more vulnerable to future attempts at blackmail. And, of course, they were very time-consuming and prevented me from getting on with real work.

On two occasions, I was telephoned by people asking for such a favour who claimed that they were acting on behalf of Kurt Waldheim, the then-president of the republic, who had famously suffered a mysterious case of retrograde amnesia in relation to his own activities during the Nazi era. By that time, weary of these intrigues, I had installed a tape-recorder on my telephone. Recording your telephone calls was illegal in Austria, which I found hilarious, given the pervasiveness of corruption in that culture: if you want to perpetrate some illegal activity, what better way of ensuring that you will not be caught in the act than declaring illegal the most effective means of proving that such an offence had occurred?

But then again, I shouldn't have been surprised: in a way, Kurt Waldheim was the trump card in Viennese poker games. One day, I was asked to lend my academic support to a strange sort of wellness centre which was run by someone using the title of Professor. When I met the man, I was told he was an old friend of Waldheim. Apparently the friendship had been formed during the war—which might have explained why this man was awarded the title of Professor despite never having been to any university. I was given to understand that giving my support would be much appreciated by Waldheim, which,

in turn, would oil the administrative machinery of university
life.

Despite the annoyance they caused, I had to admit that some
of those intrigues were almost elegant in their own warped,
peculiar way. An ambitious doctor from my team wanted to do
a PhD—not so much because he was interested in or particularly good at science but because this higher degree was the
precondition for eventually progressing towards a full professorship. Unfortunately, his research was of such poor quality
that, even with the very best connections, it was unlikely to be
deemed sufficient for a PhD. The chair of the committee
charged with evaluating the thesis seemed to owe the candidate
a favour or two and was therefore willing to close both eyes,
hold his nose and pass it regardless of its quality. Yet the work
was so poor that the other committee members seemed
unwilling to cooperate with his intention. The solution to this
problem was, of course, a clever little intrigue: the candidate
plotted with the chair to write an anonymous letter to the
committee. The letter expressed in no uncertain terms an open
threat that, if this dismal research were to be awarded a PhD,
the letter-writer would inform the press, thus prompting a
public scandal. At the next committee meeting, the chair read
out the anonymous letter to the amazed panel. Then he said,
"We all know that this thesis is not very good and we are not in
the habit of passing shoddy science. But now we have no choice.
We cannot succumb to anonymous letters blackmailing us. All
things considered, I am afraid, we have to pass the candidate."
After some discussion, our good doctor got his PhD. The
general feeling in Vienna later was that, considering the
elegance of his double bluff, he had deserved this distinction.

But the truth was that the more I got side-tracked by nonsense of this nature, the less time I had to do any meaningful
work, even though heaven knows there would have been
plenty to do. We had re-started our research into blood rheology and, in addition, we were conducting clinical trials of
various alternative therapies including homeopathy, massage,
autogenic training and acupuncture. We also had a fully

equipped motion-analysis laboratory and many other hugely expensive pieces of equipment. Money was never in short supply; the sad thing, however, was that, more often than not, it was wasted on would-be-researchers with few skills and even less motivation.

Considering these obstacles, my team did quite well; the findings of our research were reported at conferences and published in good medical journals. We also took it upon ourselves to organize numerous international conferences. During my four years in Vienna, we managed to convene well over a dozen scientific meetings. In addition, I had founded my second medical journal — *The European Journal of Physical Medicine and Rehabilitation*.

Then there was the task of teaching. As one of the largest departments of the medical school, we were expected to pull our weight and run a full programme of lectures. Oddly enough, medical students in Vienna rarely attended courses. But this little detail was irrelevant; the lectures had to go ahead, students or no students. In addition, our own staff needed to be instructed in a variety of areas: research methodology, critical thinking, clinical skills, etc.

By far the biggest part of my job, however, was to ensure a smoothly running clinical service to the rest of the 2000-bed hospital. For this purpose, we eventually employed around 100 therapists, mainly physiotherapists, occupational therapists and massage therapists. In addition, we ran several busy out-patient clinics including those for musculoskeletal conditions, stroke, cardiovascular problems, etc. Close to my heart, we even started one specifically for treating the complex health problems of the many musicians in Vienna. (The town is full of musicians who frequently suffer from work-related illnesses due to the often extreme stress that is endemic in this profession.) If nothing else, this activity provided us with an ample supply of free tickets for usually superb concerts.

To say I was busy would be an understatement. Far too busy, I felt, to start earning piles of extra money by attending patients on the Golden Mile, although I was invited several times to do such private work. This was, of course, tempting — after all, I had been told that this is where all full professors earned their money. Yet I repeatedly declined to go down this route. My decision was puzzling to many observers. Whenever asked why I would not follow the example of my colleagues, I replied that, in my view, the duties of a professor would take a hundred per cent of his time. This, of course, implied that my colleagues, who would regularly desert the university premises around lunchtime, were not doing their job properly. I imagine that such a statement did not endear me to them and suspect that gradually I was perceived as an outsider — and a potentially dangerous one — who would not play along the time-tested lines which had served everyone so very nicely for so long.

Superficially, the atmosphere amongst the 400 or so professorial colleagues was mostly cordial, but beneath the surface it was often guarded and somewhat tense. The reason, of course, was that everyone had to constantly watch his or her own back. One never quite knew whether a "kindly chat" over a cup of coffee was what it appeared to be, or whether it was an attempt to learn a few valuable details that would soon be used profitably to start a new intrigue.

I remember being invited to dinner at a colleague's home. "Very informal", he had stressed. Arriving slightly late for the occasion, I saw a room full of professors all dressed in black tie. "Informal, my foot", I thought, darkly. As I looked around, nobody returned my smile. They clearly did not approve of my distinctly casual outfit. Finally a gentleman, dressed like all the others in a black dinner jacket, caught my eye in a friendly welcoming manner. I made my way towards him hoping to have found someone to talk to, shook his hand enthusiastically and introduced myself. To my surprise he answered, "I am pleased to meet you too, and what can I get you to drink?" I had just introduced myself to the waiter hired to serve us that evening.

Social life in Vienna was often tricky. Danielle and I were invited frequently but, more often than not, only to discover that such invitations had a hidden agenda. Usually our host wanted a favour, or he wanted to enlist my participation in some elaborate plot against another colleague. Almost invariably, people were irritatingly self-important. The Germans are by no means the least pompous people in the world, so I was well used to this sort of thing, yet when it comes to pomposity the Austrians are capable of out-doing the Germans any time.

As I had the only chair of Rehabilitation Medicine in the country, the officers of the Austrian Society of Rehabilitation Medicine — not an internationally important organization by any means — were keen to get me involved in their activities. I was wined and dined by them, flattered and courted. I noticed with disbelief that they addressed their current chair as "Herr President", and with even greater incredulity that he seemed to enjoy being addressed by this ponderous title. When they had decided that I should be their next leader, I politely but firmly declined the invitation. I did not think that I would have been able keep a straight face being called Herr President.

Even though I seemed most of the time to be swimming strenuously against the tide, the first two years in Vienna were by no means all bad. They certainly brought some successes on a professional level. I had managed to set up a well-organized system that rendered an efficient service to the fast-growing number of patients in the new hospital. As the other departments of the medical school moved into the new building, our workload, and with it our staff, grew rapidly. I was proud to have coped with all these organizational and administrative tasks, and besides, I had learned many new skills that might one day come in handy. But that said, after about two years the excitement of the new challenge had palled and I found that I had begun to settle into a rather repetitive routine.

Throughout my life, I have found the experience of any type of routine a rather dangerous thing. To me, routine is the enemy of innovation and more often than not turns out to be the predecessor of boredom. My daily work increasingly became that of an administrator. I had always disliked administrative work and remained more than a little suspicious of administrators. In the setting of a medical school, administrators tend to forget that their remit should be to facilitate the work of the doctors, scientists and other health professionals. Yet, all too often, they seem to think that it should work the opposite way: everyone else should bend to their demands and work towards their purpose. In Vienna, administration became the dominant feature of my professional life—and inexorably I felt myself beginning to get frustrated with it.

In the recent past, I had oscillated between my role as a clinician and that of a scientist and had tried to achieve a balance between the two. Now I found myself increasingly hijacked by administrative demands. I had plenty of responsibility but less and less occasion to do what I would call "real" work. Somewhat to my surprise, I missed my research more than I missed the clinical practice. Several attempts to return more actively to research were blocked by not allowing us more laboratory space. The medical faculty had hired me primarily because of my scientific credentials but now they foremost wanted me to administer a smooth-running service and leave the science to other departments. But for many of my colleagues, science was not so much a calling or an urge to solve medical questions as it was a means to acquire gravitas, to varnish their curricula vitae and present themselves in a more prestigious light.

The way I saw it, I could either accept what I had on my plate and do my best to survive the game of endless intrigues and boring administration, or I could chuck it all in and start afresh elsewhere. Trusted friends with whom I discussed my situation unanimously agreed: it would be foolish to throw all this away. "Stay where you are, make the best of it. Change the system from within." This sounded entirely reasonable, but I doubted that I would be able to accomplish that task. The system was entrenched and all-powerful: if I stayed in Vienna, I would not succeed in changing the system. Instead, the system would slowly but inexorably change me.

This was a truly frightening thought. I did not want to become like the people whom I had gradually come to despise. Luckily I had Danielle: I could always discuss these issues with her, and she always understood me completely. I was only 42 — far too young to bury my dreams. For all that staying in Vienna offered me, the chance of earning loads of money and leading a life of luxury, to continue living this way would be like being locked in a golden cage. We both decided that this was not for us.

But the golden cage was locked rather more firmly than we had anticipated. Indeed, it seemed impossible to escape from it. As far as I could ascertain, none of my colleagues at the level of full professor had ever managed to voluntarily leave their position: the only exceptions were the Jewish professors who left the faculty in 1938, and they certainly had not done so voluntarily. As time passed, my frustration with this situation began to grow into desperation.

On the professional level, my particular concern was that we were unable to conduct more research. In rehabilitation medicine we used many treatments that had never been properly evaluated. Quite a few of the routinely used treatments would be considered alternative medicine in other countries: spinal manipulation, massage therapy, relaxation techniques or acupuncture, for instance. Evidence-based medicine was still an alien concept in this field. It was obvious to me that, if these treatments were to continue being widely used, they must first be shown to have a scientifically sound underpinning. I made many attempts to get this idea across, for instance, within the Austrian Society of Rehabilitation Medicine or my own medical faculty, and to be fair several research projects did eventually take off as a result of my lobbying. Yet I often suspected that they were conducted for the wrong reasons: people seemed to feel that "a bit of research" might be helpful for their attempts to climb up a few decisive steps on the career ladder. This type of motivation for conducting research seemed endemic in Vienna. To employ science principally in the service of self-advancement invites all sorts of problems, ranging from mediocrity to outright fraud. The only sound motivation to pursue research is the wish to find the truth regardless of where it may lead.

***

Danielle and I had always loved England—understandably perhaps, after all, this was where we had first met and this is where we once had been so very happy. Indeed, during our time in Munich, we had even bought a little holiday cottage in East Anglia. This is where we now tended to retreat to whenever the frustration with Vienna became difficult to bear. We talked and dreamed endlessly about going back to England, not just as tourists and solace-seekers but permanently, as residents, living and working there, making a life together in that peaceable environment which we remembered so well from our London days; an environment where outward appearances were unimportant and eccentricity raised no eyebrows.

One day in 1992, when Danielle had already gone ahead to prepare the cottage for a holiday and I was therefore left alone in Vienna, I saw the following advertisement in *The New Scientist*.

UNIVERSITY
of
EXETER

LAING CHAIR IN COMPLEMENTARY MEDICINE

Applications are invited from registered medical practitioners who have an established record for this new Chair endowed by the Maurice Laing Foundation. As Britain's first professorial appointment in the subject, the post is intended to provide an academic focus for the growing interest in the interface between orthodox and complementary medicine.

The successful candidate, who will be based in the University's well established Centre for Complementary Health Studies, will be required to develop research into the techniques and effectiveness of the various branches of complementary medicine, to encourage the assimilation of appropriate complementary techniques into orthodox medicine, and to engage in teaching. The appointment will be for ten years in the first instance.

Details from Personnel, University of Exeter, Exeter EX4 4QJ; (0392) 263100 or e.mail Personnel@uk.ac.exeter. Closing date 13 October 1992.

It seemed tailor made for me. Here was an opportunity to bring the skills of a scientist to bear on an area of medicine that at that time had scarcely seen any serious research. All the disparate paths I had taken during my professional life seemed to converge here.

At this stage, I had been quietly working on research into alternative medicine for some time. My main research interest was still blood rheology but every now and then the many research questions that had been raised during my time at the homeopathic hospital came back to me. Whenever I had the opportunity during the years that followed, I had tried to address some of them. In this way, I had accumulated a small portfolio of around 30 research articles related to alternative medicine — a modest portfolio compared to my publications in other areas, maybe, but still a good start. I instantly phoned Danielle in Suffolk and we discussed the possibility animatedly. There was no hesitation whatsoever: I simply had to apply.

When, a few weeks later, an invitation to attend an interview arrived, Danielle and I were as excited as little children. I suspected that my chances were slim; most likely the post had already been earmarked for someone else. I knew only too well that this is often the case in academia, and somehow the Exeter post looked as though the race had been decided before the starting shot had been fired. Yet, if nothing else, this was going to be an interesting trip to a part of England that we did not know well.

The vetting process for the Exeter post was a very British affair. It started in the late afternoon with a sherry party and plenty of small talk with a confusing array of people in pin-striped suits. All the short-listed candidates, the entire interview panel and several other luminaries of Exeter had been invited. In the evening, there was a semi-formal dinner along similar lines. It made me smile to think that the British equivalent of the ponderous system of public lectures that characterized the Austrian vetting procedure was merely an informal chit-chat.

Next morning, there were interviews for each candidate. Mine lasted less than an hour. Each of the panel members asked one or two questions. The panel consisted of about eight senior university staff and two external advisors, both of whom were physicians: one was a former Surgeon General of the British Navy and the other one was the Queen's homeopath.

My fears had been correct: the post had indeed been earmarked for one particular candidate. The panel, however, seemed pleasantly surprised by my application. None of the other candidates had previously occupied a senior position and none had extensive experience in basic and clinical research as well as in clinical medicine and teaching. I had been in two professorial posts in two different countries and had conducted research in a number of different medical fields. In addition, I was a clinician as well as a scientist. Finally, I had hands-on experience with several alternative therapies both as a practitioner as well as an investigator.

To my delight, the panel felt that I was a serious contender, but at the same time they appeared mystified by my wish to leave my current prestigious and far superior post in Vienna. Their suspicion was, as I learnt later, that I merely wanted to secure the University of Exeter job offer in order to re-negotiate the terms of my current position in Vienna. This sort of thing does happen quite regularly in academia, and there was a chance that I was playing this game too. For several months, the University thus continued to negotiate both with me and with the candidate who had previously been their favourite. I also met Sir Maurice Laing, who had endowed the chair, and made further visits to Exeter. At one stage, the Exeter Vice-Chancellor even phoned Danielle in Vienna: "Are you sure you and your husband want to move to Exeter?", he asked her. "Quite sure", she replied. Eventually, after an agonizing wait, the appointment panel was able to reach a decision: they offered me the job.

The door of the golden cage had been opened. Jubilant, unable to believe our good fortune, we fled.

Chapter 4

Mission Impossible

On 17 September 1993, we arrived in Exeter with two huge lorries full of our furniture and other belongings. We had bought a slightly dilapidated yet rather splendid old house in the centre of Exeter. The builders had promised that the much-needed renovations would be finished before our arrival but, as happens with builders everywhere, that had unfortunately been an over-optimistic prediction. For the first three or four weeks we lived in total chaos, yet despite the thick clouds of plaster dust, mountains of rubble and treacherous voids left by pried-up floorboards, we were utterly euphoric. Nothing could possibly spoil our excitement: we had arrived amongst people we liked and felt instantly comfortable with. As soon as the head of the postgraduate medical school, Prof. Perreira-Gray, learned that we had arrived, he called with a bottle of champagne to celebrate the occasion with us: what kindness and what style! This, we felt, was the way to live and the place to be.

The first few months in Exeter were dominated by an over-whelming sense of relief and profound happiness: we had finally managed to make our home in the country of our dreams; we felt like two refugees who had found their way to freedom.

People seemed both fascinated and puzzled by us. What had brought us here? How could we possibly have chosen the staid, unassuming country town of Exeter in preference to the sophis-tication and the bright lights of Vienna? How could anyone in his right mind exchange the medical school of Vienna with a mere postgraduate medical centre in Exeter? My short, and truthful, answer usually was: "We truly love England and are more than happy to be here." Most people were very pleased, even flattered with this explanation but, of course, it was more complicated than that. Yes, we had long dreamt of living in England, and yes, I desperately wanted to escape the politely suffocating, intrigue-ridden world of Viennese academic medicine. But I also wanted to turn my full attention back to research, and the Exeter appointment offered a wonderful opportunity to do just that. I had never forgotten my years in the earnest collegial atmosphere of St George's, which was in many ways so singularly British and so unlike the research environments that I had subsequently experienced. And then there was the nature of the research itself: I would have been content researching almost any area that I knew well enough to investigate competently, but the fact that this appointment was focused on research into alternative medicine seemed particularly intriguing to me. I was going to investigate uncharted territory — and what could be more exciting than that?

Alternative medicine had by then begun to attract a considerable amount of public attention — and not a little controversy. To me, raised as I had been in Germany, where alternative medicine had been considered unremarkable, just another ancillary means of supporting general health, the passions that could be so quickly aroused by this subject in other countries such as the UK and the US were philosophically and culturally intriguing. It seemed that now was an ideal time to shine the cool, dispassionate light of reason onto the whole topic of alternative medicine, to evaluate scientifically what its contribution had been to date, and to establish what role it might conceivably play in the age of evidence-based medicine.

I had no idea just how deeply emotional and worryingly politicized the debates in and around alternative medicine had already become, but I was about to find out.

As my new position was the first chair of its kind, the university administrators had decided to organize a press conference. Universities tend to like such events: they create publicity — and publicity would create prestige which might in turn generate funds. I was not unfamiliar with the task of facing the press and knew that these occasions could easily turn awkward: one can never predict what questions journalists might come up with. In this particular instance, not only I but also Sir Maurice Laing (who had endowed the chair) as well as the Vice Chancellor of the University were to make brief statements, after which the journalists would have the opportunity to quiz us. As alternative medicine was a controversial topic, we tried to play it safe: the Vice Chancellor praised the generosity of Sir Maurice and spoke of the unique opportunity his endowment would offer for both the University and the field of complementary medicine, as well as of the University's good fortune in finding an experienced professor to tackle this difficult and important task. For his part, Sir Maurice told the audience of his deep conviction that rigorous research and proper science were the best ways to reveal the true value of the treatments that he and his wife had repeatedly found helpful.

Then it was my turn. I briefly outlined my professional background, explained what rigorous research in alternative medicine would entail and where it might take us. When I had finished, one journalist in the front row raised his hand: "What will you do, Prof Ernst, when your medical colleagues turn out to be sceptical about alternative medicine?" Shooting from the hip, I answered: "I am not worried about that, because I intend to be more sceptical than they are." As soon as these words had crossed my lips, I wondered how the benefactor would take this somewhat provocative and unexpected comment. My concern turned out to be unfounded: everybody smiled approvingly, including Sir Maurice, probably thinking that I had not meant it entirely seriously — but indeed I had.

A considerably more aggressive and curious public challenge occurred a few weeks later during a conference hosted by the Research Council for Complementary Medicine in London. This organization had been established a few years earlier with the aim of conducting and facilitating research in all areas of alternative medicine. My impression of this institution, and indeed of the various other groups operating in this area, was that they were far too uncritical, and often proved to be hopelessly biased in favour of alternative medicine. This, I thought, was an extraordinary phenomenon: should research councils and similar bodies not have a duty to be critical and be primarily concerned about the quality of the research rather than the overall tenor of the results? Should research not be critical by nature? In this regard, alternative medicine appeared to be starkly different from any other type of health care I had encountered previously.

On short notice, I had accepted an invitation to address this meeting packed with about 100 proponents of alternative medicine. I felt that their enthusiasm and passion were charming but, no matter whom I talked to, there seemed to be little or no understanding of the role of science in all this. A strange naïvety pervaded this audience: alternative practitioners and their supporters seemed a bit like children playing "doctor and patient". The language, the rituals and the façade were all more or less in place, but somehow they seemed strangely detached from reality. It felt a bit as though I had landed on a different planet. The delegates passionately wanted to promote alternative medicine, while I, with equal passion and conviction, wanted to conduct good science. The two aims were profoundly different. Nevertheless, I managed to convince myself that they were not irreconcilable, and that we would manage to combine our passions and create something worthwhile, perhaps even groundbreaking.

Everyone was excited about the new chair in Exeter; high hopes and expectations filled the room. The British alternative medicine scene had long felt discriminated against because they had no academic representation to speak of. I certainly did sympathize with this particular aspect and felt assured that, essentially, I was amongst friends who realized that my expertise and their enthusiasm could add up to bring about progress for the benefit of many patients.

During my short speech, I summarized my own history as a physician and a scientist and outlined what I intended to do in my new post — nothing concrete yet, merely the general gist. I stressed that my plan was to apply science to this field in order to find out what works and what doesn't; what is safe and what isn't. Science, I pointed out, generates progress through asking critical questions and through testing hypotheses. Alternative medicine would either be shown by good science to be of value, or it would turn out to be little more than a passing fad. The endowment of the Laing chair represented an important milestone on the way towards the impartial evaluation of alternative medicine, and surely this would be in the best interest of all parties concerned.

To me, all this seemed an entirely reasonable approach, particularly as it merely reiterated what I had just published in an editorial for *The Lancet* entitled "Scrutinizing the Alternatives".

My audience, however, was not impressed. When I had finished, there was a stunned, embarrassed silence. Finally someone shouted angrily from the back row: "How did they dare to appoint a doctor to this chair?" I was startled by this question and did not quite understand. What had prompted this reaction? What did this audience expect? Did they think my qualifications were not good enough? Why were they upset by the appointment of a doctor? Who else, in their view, might be better equipped to conduct medical research?

It wasn't until weeks later that it dawned on me: they had been waiting for someone with a strong commitment to the promotion of alternative medicine. Such a commitment could only come from an alternative practitioner. A doctor personified the establishment, and "alternative" foremost symbolized "anti-establishment". My little speech had upset them because it confirmed their worst fears of being annexed by "the establishment". These enthusiasts had hoped for a believer from their own ranks and certainly not for a doctor-scientist to be appointed to the world's first chair of complementary medicine. They had expected that Exeter University would lend its support to their commercial and ideological interests; they had little understanding of the concept that universities should not be in the business of promoting anything other than high standards.

Even today, after having given well over 600 lectures on the topic of alternative medicine, and after coming on the receiving end of ever more hostile attacks, aggressive questions and personal insults, this particular episode is still etched deeply into my memory. In a very real way, it set the scene for the two decades to come: the endless conflicts between my agenda of testing alternative medicine scientifically and the fervent aspirations of enthusiasts to promote alternative medicine uncritically. That our positions would prove mutually incompatible had been predictable from the very start. The writing had been on the wall — but it took me a while to be able to fully understand the message.

***

In contrast to Germany or Austria, alternative medicine in the UK is not normally in the hands of doctors. Instead, it is practised by a disparate array of independent workers — acupuncturists, chiropractors, homeopaths, herbalists, reflexologists, aromatherapists, naturopaths, healers, iridologists, massage therapists, osteopaths, etc. These alternative practitioners have not studied medicine; in fact, many have little training and no medical or academic education to speak of.

What is worse, most alternative practitioners exhibit a deep resentment towards science. By its very definition, "alternative" signifies "anti-establishment" and, in turn, this is understood as "anti-science". Being both a doctor and a scientist, I was the perfect symbol of the establishment: in the eyes of a fundamentalist I embodied "THE ENEMY", someone who must be resisted, fought and eventually defeated — or at the very least silenced.

But, of course, it is in the British national character to abide by the rules of fair play: it would be very poor form to deny the new professor his chance. Thus open hostilities were postponed and, for two or three years, the world of alternative medicine seemed to hold its breath, giving me the benefit of the doubt.

Meanwhile, both my work and I were watched with great suspicion; my aims, methods and research concepts were questioned, and aspersions were none too subtly cast on my motives and integrity.

Being constantly challenged in this way was not at all a problem for me; on the contrary, after the stuffily devote atmosphere in Vienna, I found it quite stimulating and continued to harbour the hope that it might be possible to harness the criticism in a constructive way. After all, my team and I were about to venture into uncharted territory, and it was therefore necessary and potentially helpful to make sure that each step was carefully considered.

I was keenly aware of the concerns and worries of alternative practitioners and ready to accommodate them as much as I possibly could. Consequently, I accepted every invitation to give lectures and regularly spent long hours in discussions and debates trying to make sure that all reasonable views were taken on board. However, what did eventually tire, and at times really exasperated me, was the insistence of many in the alternative medicine camp that their favoured therapy should somehow be exempt from scientific testing.

Actually, it was often even more extreme than that. Many players in the UK alternative medicine scene also rejected the concepts and the tools of mainstream medicine. Most alternative practitioners felt no need to question, let alone test, their traditions, ideas, notions or claims. Those few who would consider science at all would advocate it as a means of proving that their concepts were correct, usually with a view to improving their status, advancing their trade or increasing their income. The field of alternative medicine seemed rife with fundamentalists; people who had an evangelical conviction; crackpots who could not think straight; garrulous pseudo-researchers who had never conducted real research or even tried to understand science; pseudoscientists who found it not unusual to research an entirely implausible treatment and produce one false-positive result after the other; and overt anti-scientists who believed that science was a serious threat to everything they believed in. Unfortunately, such attitudes turned out to be right at my doorstep, and I had to address them sooner and more directly than I had ever imagined.

***

The University of Exeter had received the initial Laing endowment of £1.5 million not least because, a few years earlier, the University had opened the Centre for Complementary Health Studies (CCHS). Negotiations between the Laing representatives and other (arguably more prestigious) institutions to accept the endowment had failed, apparently because these other universities feared that a chair in complementary medicine might tarnish their academic reputation. From today's perspective this seems hard to imagine but, in the early 1990s, things were very different: alternative medicine was still seen as a subject too dubious to be allowed into the "ivory tower of academia".

Without wanting or even realizing it, I had become the director of the CCHS. I had not appreciated that this role would automatically fall into my lap: the job description had merely stated that I would be "based" at the centre. Taking charge of it meant that I had unknowingly ousted the centre's two former co-directors — and not only that: I had become their new boss. The two ex-directors, the herbalist Simon Mills and the acupuncturist Roger Hill, seemed distinctly miffed at this turn of events and appeared to feel uneasy at the prospect of someone breathing down their neck.

It occurred to me that I had landed myself in a rather awkward situation. For the time being, I thought it would be prudent to interfere as little as possible with any of the activities at the CCHS. I decided to lie low for a few months and simply observe what this unit was all about.

What I learnt in the course of this period worried — no, it horrified — me. I had become the head of a small group responsible for teaching a Bachelor of Science (BSc) course tailor-made for alternative practitioners. In order to judge the quality of the course and the thoroughness of student supervision, I studied a dozen theses that had been written by the centre's former graduates and had earned them the desired BSc degree. My hope was to see whether any of this material might be publishable. This would have been a good way to put the CCHS on the map of medical research and, at the same time, it might reward the students for their hard work. As it turned out, none of these documents would have, in my view, passed the process of peer-review in a reputable medical journal. I had read lots of poor research in my life, but when it came to pseudoscience and inadequate research these documents seemed in a class of their own. The typical thesis would be based on a small survey of the student's own patients who had elected to use a particular therapy and were evidently happy with their choice—otherwise they would hardly have continued paying for it. The student would pose a few questions to the patients about the perceived value of the intervention. Predictably, the answers were extremely positive. Thus the conclusion of this "research" might be that this particular treatment modality—aromatherapy, for example—was clearly effective and should be used more widely. Perhaps I am exaggerating a bit, but the point is clear: this type of enquiry would tell us nothing more instructive about the worth of a treatment than the observation that, if people choose to pay for something, they tend to claim that they have spent their money well.

Things quickly got worse when someone told me about the "Feasibility Study" which Exeter University had submitted to Sir Maurice Laing in order to compete for the endowment. The day I managed to obtain a copy of this document, I needed a very stiff drink to relax. To my shock and horror, the study described the role of the new chair essentially as designing and running more educational courses to bachelor and masters level using various means, including distance learning. This had certainly not been my intention, and neither was it the remit I had signed up to.

In truth, while all my previous jobs had entailed some teaching commitments, teaching was not an aspect of my work that I truly enjoyed. I had always been acutely aware of my own shortcomings as a teacher: the memory of the uninspiring teachers of my childhood, whose only reason for remaining in that profession seemed to be the malign pleasure they derived from exercising power over their reluctant pupils, had left an indelible impression on me. But, most of all, I was eager now to spend the majority of my time doing research. In other words, teaching alternative practitioners was neither my calling nor my skill; on the contrary, it seemed a bit like the subject of a nightmare. So I went straight to the Vice Chancellor, David Harrison, to discuss this issue with him directly.

During my two decades in Exeter, I had the opportunity to work under three different Vice Chancellors. David Harrison, the first one, was a true gentleman, a compliment that, unfortunately, I would hesitate to pay to his two successors. He smiled and assured me not to worry: of course, he knew about my plans to concentrate on rigorous research and he fully supported it. Not only that, but he was very clear about the fact that the University had appointed me precisely because of my research ability and track record in science. The "Feasibility Study" should be ignored, he said. What a relief!

But what was I to do with the CCHS and its two ex-directors? The more I learnt about their BSc course, the more concerned I became. In addition to some solid and well-taught subjects such as statistics and law, which were in the hands of respectable professionals recruited from other university departments, students were exposed to what I felt was a steady stream of pseudoscience about energy healing, vitalism, traditional Chinese medicine, homeopathy, etc., all taught by naïvely uncritical believers in the respective subjects. How on earth could I take responsibility for such an irrational curriculum?

What was I to do? My alarm-bells were ringing loud and clear, even keeping me awake at night. A BSc course in claptrap and my agenda of rigorous scientific enquiry were as incompatible as fire and water. With the best will in the world, this story could not possibly have a happy ending. I had started my contract in October 1993, and by the end of that year I had realized that the CCHS was a disaster waiting to happen. It had the potential to impede my research agenda and even to seriously tarnish my academic career, as well as the reputation of Exeter University.

On arrival in Exeter, I had been elated. Only two months later, my enthusiasm had been replaced by grinding worry. There were moments when I started to doubt that leaving Vienna had been the right decision. This sentiment of having made a wrong professional move was entirely new to me. Of course, I had felt a strong need to escape the stultifying environ-ment of Vienna with its "golden cage" but even there I never had experienced deep regrets. In Vienna, I had been in charge of about 120 staff, in a well-funded department that was housed in very large and brand new premises. In Exeter, by contrast, I found myself with less than a handful of recalcitrant co-workers, no rooms to speak of and tightly limited funds. I had given up a professorship for life and accepted one with an uncertain long-term future. I had halved my salary and had swapped a luxury office for one that looked more like a broom cupboard. I had exchanged a whole armada of secretaries for one singularly ungifted temp. Worst of all, I had come here to conduct research in conjunction with alternative practitioners who, on closer inspection, seemed to feel threatened by science in general and me in particular.

Why did you take this job? I asked myself. How on earth can you sort out this mess? All I had wanted was to lead a peaceful and quiet life in England, to get away from the academic in-fighting in Vienna, to be out of the limelight and do some meaningful research. I hadn't specifically sought out alternative medicine research. Yes, it was an interesting subject, but there were many other topics that were at least as fascinating.

Ruefully I remembered how most of my friends had warned me that a move into alternative medicine might turn out to be a perfect way to ruin a promising academic career. I had ignored them, not least because I did not want a "career" in the first place. I had happily decided to retire from my Viennese life as an academic high-flyer, and I certainly did not wish to fight against anyone anymore. The last months in Vienna had been a long, unpleasant battle with an increasing number of adversaries; not being a born fighter, this struggle had worn me out. Now I was looking for a calm environment in which to research productively. Had I gone from the frying pan into the fire?

What on earth could I do? It seemed to me that there was no other solution than to roll up my sleeves and get on with the job at hand. The only way I could accomplish anything, I decided, was to completely detach myself from the CCHS and its odd-balls, and if at all possible to do so in a way that did not create too much fuss or ill feeling. I quickly negotiated this option with the appropriate university officials who proved surprisingly sympathetic to my suggestion. It felt a bit like forcing doors that had already been open: everyone I talked to saw my point and promised to support my plans.

My next task was to consult the two external advisors to my chair concerning the need for separation from the CCHS. The Laing Foundation had appointed Dr William Davey, the Queen's homeopath, to guide my actions, and the University had asked Sir James Watt, retired Surgeon General of the British Navy, to act as their advisor. I was not at all sure where these two individuals might stand regarding the CCHS. Davey in particular seemed to identify with the idea of promoting homeopathy to a degree that worried me. It therefore took some careful preparatory work followed by gentle persuasion. But eventually both advisors agreed that, in order to build up a high quality research team and an international reputation for first class research, I needed be freed of the shackles of the CCHS.

Then I had to convince the two former co-directors of the CCHS that it would be in their best interest to consent to the separation. This last step in my plan turned out to be a piece of cake: when I offered them £50,000 of the Laing endowment (as had been agreed with my peers) together with the prospect of regaining their independence from me, they could barely hide their excitement. They were clearly delighted with the thought of once again being in charge and able to continue their forays into quackery. They accepted my proposition without any hesitation whatsoever.

This was perhaps less surprising than it looked: by that time, our relations had become fairly tense. In my frustration concerning the academic standards of the CCHS I had gone as far as to declare that "this is a university, not a knitting class". They did not consider my comment to be funny at all and made sure it became widely known around the campus and misunderstood as a sexist remark. Luckily I was able to point out that knitting is not necessarily an exclusively female occupation and that assuming otherwise was arguably sexist in itself. This and many other disagreements had created an atmosphere of overt animosity between us. Consequently, they seemed as happy to get rid of me as I was delighted to move on. About two years later, the CCHS was closed down—although not because of its promotion of anti-science, pseudoscience and outright quackery, nor because of its undistinguished academic standards, but for the more prosaic reason that its directors had failed to render it financially viable.

Roughly a decade later, a lively debate emerged about what had by then had become sardonically known as "quackademia" —first on a national, and eventually also international, level. At that stage, numerous university courses in alternative medicine had sprung up, as far as I could see, all of them dominated by pseudoscientists. Eventually, alarm at the teaching of quackery at university level began to grow. An increasing number of experts felt that it was wrong, even dangerous, to brainwash youngsters with mystical nonsense, potentially undermining rationality and critical thinking in the larger society. As a consequence, most of these alternative medicine courses were closed down again. I pride myself on being among the very first to achieve such a victory of reason, without undue fuss, controversy or publicity.

The first major obstacle on the road to some proper science had been overcome. Now I needed to organize the logistical infrastructure for successful research: a team of bright and dedicated co-workers, adequate premises — and, of course, money to pay for all this.

Dr Karl-Ludwig Resch had been my co-worker ever since he had graduated from medical school in Munich and started working as my research assistant in the field of blood rheology. Later, he had followed me from Germany to Austria and, in 1993, he volunteered to come to Exeter. He had done a splendid job in helping my Viennese team get organized, and had been particularly useful in encouraging critical thinking among our co-workers. We had even managed to establish a course on this important topic in the Viennese medical curriculum.

Now, once again, Dr Resch proved to be an invaluable help in setting up a research team. We became close friends and our work continued to be successful — so successful, in fact, that after only one and a half years in Exeter he was offered a professorship back in Germany which he accepted and holds to the present day. Other researchers followed, most notably Dr Adrian White, an experienced and nationally known acupuncturist. Within a year of our arrival in Exeter, my team had grown into a group of a handful of co-workers with expertise in a range of relevant areas and, most importantly, with lots of enthusiasm for giving "mission impossible" a good try.

My next step was to find adequate premises for my growing unit. This unfortunately proved more of an obstacle than anticipated. For several months, we were shunted from one provisional location to the next. At one time, the university administration even tried to squeeze us into a Portakabin. This was where I drew the line and protested forcefully. Eventually suitable rooms were rented close to the Postgraduate Medical School (PGMS), which, a few years later, developed into the Peninsula Medical School (PMS). Even though my contract was with the University rather than the medical school *per se*, I had always been keen to be affiliated as closely as possible with my medical colleagues. The director of the PGMS, Prof Pereira-Gray, was most supportive of this aim, yet despite his influence, I was unable to get rooms on the hospital grounds. It seemed that some colleagues wanted nothing to do with anyone related to alternative medicine: the idea of a "witch doctor" amongst their ranks made them feel uneasy, it was rumoured. This attitude only changed once the separation between the CCHS and my research unit had become general knowledge and after the generally sceptical hospital consultants had read some of my early articles, finally convincing them that my aim was not to promote but to scientifically investigate alternative treatments.

The final item on my "to do" list was money. The initial Laing endowment of £1.5 million was certainly generous but it was not nearly enough to support a sufficiently sizable research team for any length of time. Essentially, the financial plan was for my unit to live off the income that the invested capital would generate. In order to build up a strong team I therefore had to find more money. The university fundraiser was charged with spearheading this effort; after all, the University had signed a contract with Sir Maurice Laing to match his funding.

We decided to hold regular discussion meetings about how to raise the necessary funds. Even though our attempts to procure funding met with little success, I was repeatedly assured that, if all else failed, we would be underwritten from the University's substantial core endowment. University officials made it very clear that they viewed this issue to be a priority.

From the start, it was obvious to me that money was the Achilles heel of the whole undertaking, but as far as I could see there was no choice but to trust the many assurances my peers were giving me: funding would be found by hook or by crook. This trust would prove misplaced.

***

Over the years I had acquired considerable expertise in the design and conducting of clinical trials. I had run and published about two dozen such investigations and I was certain that this type of research would be the most productive way to evaluate alternative medicine. The original advertisement for my post had described the task of the new professor as "encouraging the assimilation of appropriate treatments into conventional medicine". As I saw it, the best possible way to test the effectiveness of any treatment, new or old, standard or unconventional, mainstream or alternative, was by conducting clinical trials, and everybody with whom I discussed this question—including Davey and Watt, the two external advisers—agreed with this view.

I was equally convinced that thorough investigation of the safety of alternative treatments was urgently required; in fact, the more I thought about it, the more I felt that this issue should be at the top of our priority list.

People tend to assume that so-called "natural" treatments are risk-free, yet one needs to look no further than deadly nightshade, botulism or poisonous mushrooms to illustrate that such notions about the harmlessness of nature are ill founded. Patient safety is far too important to allow it to be based on mere assumptions. What we needed were facts, not opinions. Alternativists usually disagreed with this view, pointing out that conventional medicine, and pharmaceuticals in particular, were burdened with much greater risks than alternative treatments. I argued that, while this may well be so, the worth of *any* intervention must be seen in the context of a balance between its risks and its demonstrable benefits. If the benefits are uncertain, then even relatively small risks will weigh heavily and tilt the risk–benefit balance into the negative.

As a nation, we spend huge amounts of money on alternative medicine. Globally the annual sum is now about US $100 billion, and one estimate we arrived at in cooperation with the BBC implied that, in the UK, we spent £1.6 billion each year on alternative medicine. It would therefore seem entirely prudent to investigate whether this money is well spent. Are alternative treatments cost effective? Particularly on the political level, this question seems highly relevant, especially if increasingly scarce public money and resources are to be diverted in order to pay for the use of such treatments alongside standard care. In my view this was, and remains, an important research topic and a question that still has the potential to determine the future of this field.

Our three main research questions had thus been determined:

- Efficacy

- Safety

- Cost

After roughly one year of preparatory work, everything seemed to be in place for our research to start in earnest. Around this time, I was asked to write a "mission statement" for my new research unit, which had by then been given the official title of the Department of Complementary Medicine. "A very British thing", a friend explained when I enquired what a mission statement might be. "Just put on paper what your unit stands for." I gave it some thought and formulated our mission as clearly and concisely as I could:

- To conduct rigorous, inter-disciplinary and international collaborative research into the efficacy, safety and cost of complementary medicine.

- To further analytical thinking in this area.

People reading my mission statement tended to be slightly puzzled by the inclusion of "analytical thinking" as a specific, separate item, but even after two decades, I am still pleased that I added it. The fostering of critical analysis is vital to any scientific endeavour, and perhaps particularly so in a field that, until now, has been so accustomed to special pleading and so sheltered from objective evaluation.

While studying medicine, I had not been well instructed in critical thinking. It was only later that I had realized how vulnerable health care can be without it. In Vienna, we had managed to smuggle the subject onto the medical curriculum. In Exeter, I soon discovered how woefully uncritical the attitude towards alternative medicine frequently was. This phenomenon was noticeable not just when reading the popular press or when talking to lay people but also, and perhaps even more worryingly, it was equally obvious in discussions with health care professionals. This lack of critical thinking, I felt, had the potential to hinder progress or even to cause significant harm. Particularly during the later years of my time in Exeter, the theme of critical analysis would dominate my work.

My peers were happy with the mission statement, and most rational thinkers who saw it thought it was ambitious but sound. However, in many alternative medicine enthusiasts it aroused suspicion; they seemed dismayed and felt that it was misguided. Some offered the opinion that alternative medicine should not be scientifically scrutinized at all. Others believed that my work should be directed much more at promoting alternative medicine rather than questioning it. Some argued that a professor of complementary medicine should be unabashedly sympathetic towards those working in this area, and that this attitude should be specifically articulated in any mission statement. Yet others argued that the mission statement should focus primarily on sociological or psychological issues rather than medical questions.

I listened patiently and politely to everyone who wanted to comment. I discussed, re-evaluated, re-discussed and reconsidered my position. But whichever way I looked at it, I couldn't escape the conclusion that the arguments of my critics were at best unconvincing or irrelevant, and at worst they were downright misleading—and I became determined to show why.

I was not a politician, nor was I a propagandist or an ideologue: I was simply a scientist, and as such my role was not to further the ambitions of interested parties but to determine the true value of alternative medicine. Patients and consumers have an absolute right to know the truth about the value of the treatments they frequently use, and the obligation of a researcher is to determine truth. That required a rigorous medical research agenda which would steer us clear of the postmodernist approach advocated by so many who tried to influence me and my growing team of investigators.

Over the years, my resolve to stay on this straight and narrow path of objective medical research has provoked endless criticism. Indeed, the potential for conflict had been there from the outset, when, at that very first lecture for alternative practitioners, I had been publicly challenged: "How did they dare to appoint a doctor to this chair?" Now that I had realized that this tension existed, I had to decide how to deal with it in my professional capacity.

Initially I made a conscious effort to avoid discord, not because I lacked the necessary courage or convincing arguments, but for a variety of other reasons, both personal and pragmatic. Firstly, I do not enjoy disagreements nearly as much as some people seem to think. If conflict becomes unavoidable, I can certainly put up a good fight, but that does not mean I enjoy the process. Secondly, I was honestly tired of having disputes. The battles I had fought in Vienna had left me drained and somewhat bruised. Over the years, I did develop a thicker skin but it certainly was not something I was born with. Thirdly, conflicts take far too much time, energy and concentration away from one's real work: the more time I was compelled to spend locked in combat, the less time I would have to focus on the science I was so eager to generate. Fourthly, if the worst came to the worst, and if I was going to have to defend my views at every turn, I needed to be entirely sure of my ground. Solid research was the only way to ensure that; and I felt the need to do the research first and have the arguments later.

Chapter 5

Trials and Tribulations

Research into alternative medicine differs from most other kinds of medical research in one significant way: there is a strong pre-existing element of public affection and enthusiasm for this type of health care. The rapid rise of alternative medicine during the last two decades and the increasingly insistent demands for its inclusion as a part of standard medical education have moved it from the realm of the purely therapeutic and placed it squarely into the forum of public policy. Anyone who sets out to scrutinize or test the worth of a particular alternative therapy must therefore be prepared at the outset to deal with a certain degree of lobbying by loyal adherents. Similarly, if the research produces results that are, in the minds of the adherents, equivocal or unfavourable, the researcher can expect a torrent of impassioned and often unapologetically personal criticism and attacks on the national stage.

This was something I had definitely not anticipated at the time I took up my post at Exeter. On several occasions in those early days I had expressed my inclination to begin my research work by focusing on those alternative treatments that were particularly popular in Britain. I had assumed that this would mean things like homeopathy and chiropractic, modalities that internationally occupied a very prominent place in the alternative pantheon. I certainly had never imagined that spiritual healing would be high on the list.

It came as a bit of a surprise, therefore, when I was approached by a group of spiritual healers—actually they came to my home and rang the doorbell—expressing great delight that I was interested in studying their craft. At first I was bewildered. "Why would I do that?", I asked. "Because you said so—you promised to focus on popular alternative therapies, and we are by far the largest group of alternative practitioners in the UK."

They were absolutely correct. In the early 1990s, about 14,000 healers were registered with the UK Federation of Spiritual Healers—a total larger than the number of chiropractors, osteopaths, acupuncturists, homeopaths and herbalists put together; in fact, at the time, it was almost equal to the number of physicians in general practice.

Healers believe that there is a universal "healing energy" that emanates from cosmic, divine or other supernatural sources, and that they have the power to channel this energy into the bodies of their patients. Assisted by this channelled energy, they claim, patients are able to heal themselves.

In truth, I had never planned to investigate this area, and even if I had, it would not have been a high priority. I had always been of the opinion that it would be wiser and more productive to concentrate on investigating treatments that were based on some kind of physical or biological hypothesis, and spiritual healing certainly doesn't come under that rubric. There is no way to explain logically how spiritual healing might work, based as it is on a set of beliefs and assumptions that are essentially metaphysical. That obviously makes it very much harder to design anything approaching a rigorous study. But, although dedicating research efforts towards a scientifically implausible treatment was unlikely to be a fruitful endeavour, the truth was that I had been hoisted by my own petard: after promising that I would concentrate initially on the most popular alternative therapies, I had little choice but to go forward with the design of an investigation of spiritual healing.

I began the process by applying for a grant from the Wellcome Trust, and started discussions with five local healers, trying to figure out how best to design and run a methodically sound study of this mystical therapy. The healers came highly recommended by their professional organization, which was as much of a reassurance as one could hope for that they were as good as they get. I put my initial reservations firmly aside: together, my team and I were determined to give it our best shot. If nothing else, this might be an interesting experience. As it turned out, "interesting" was an understatement.

To my surprise, our grant application was successful, and we received £50,000 to go ahead with planning a study—by no means a huge sum for a clinical trial, but it was a start. The terms of the grant were most unusual: the Wellcome Trust allowed us considerable latitude to design the trial collaboratively, drawing on the wisdom of both the healers and my research team. Not even the type of illness or medical condition that was to be the subject of spiritual healing had been predetermined.

Of necessity, our research had to rely heavily on the input of the healers themselves. They, after all, were the experts, the ones who knew best how they go about treating a certain type of patient to achieve a particular type of result. It has always struck me as important to incorporate such expertise at an early planning stage of a study. Had we not put the therapists themselves at the heart of the planning process, we would have been in danger of conducting a trial which was either entirely useless or which failed to test spiritual healing, and merely debunked it. In addition, as in any clinical trial, we required the input of methodologists with experience in the design, conduct, evaluation and publication of such investigations. If these aspects were neglected, as they often are in alternative medicine research, we might have ended up conducting a trial that failed to answer the specific research question at hand. And finally, of course, we needed to have the medical staff on board, the clinicians with expert knowledge in managing patients suffering from the condition to be treated—but in the early stages, the healers were still uncertain which type of patients they should choose.

After considerable debate, we all agreed that their best option would be to go for patients suffering from chronic pain. Our healers felt that, since they had had ample experience in treating pain and had reportedly previously seen excellent results, they would be able to relieve pain effectively in the context of the study. My team liked the idea, not least because there is never a shortage of pain patients, and we thus felt confident about recruiting sufficient numbers for an adequately sized study. Our colleagues from the local pain clinic were delighted to cooperate by providing us with their expertise in pain management and sending us their chronic pain patients. So, all the essential three areas of expertise were covered.

Next, the healers had to decide the details of the treatment schedule. They determined that no less than eight treatment sessions were required to generate a marked pain reduction. This created a bit of a problem for us: our budget was tight and, of course, the healers wanted to be paid for their services. We agreed to their demand of eight sessions but, as a consequence, there were hardly any funds left to support my team, but somehow we managed nevertheless.

From the outset, I had made it clear to everyone that the aim of our research was to test whether spiritual healing generated effects beyond a placebo response. Quite apart from the fact that this was the issue that interested me most, it also was, more importantly, the question on the basis of which we had obtained the funds from the Wellcome Trust. But what would constitute an adequate placebo intervention in a trial of spiritual healing?

When we study a drug, the placebo problem is usually quite easy to overcome: we only need to produce a pill that contains no active ingredient but is otherwise indistinguishable from the real thing. In alternative medicine, though, things are typically not quite that simple. Particularly with physical or psychological interventions, such as acupuncture or spiritual healing, there is normally no obvious placebo or sham therapy which is inert (as a placebo must be), and which patients find indistinguishable from the real treatment (which is the second precondition for an adequate placebo).

After further discussions with our five healers, we settled for actors, or "sham healers", who would masquerade as healers. They would be taught the ritual of a healing session by our healers but, not being trained healers, they would not be emitting any "healing energy" and would thus be therapeutically inert. If they followed the ritual of the healers, our patients would be unable to distinguish them from the real healers. This seemed like a perfect solution to a tricky problem, and everyone was happy to have found it.

Little did we know that a big surprise awaited us. After teaching the ritual of healing to our five actors, the healers decided that our study design was no good after all. With breathless excitement, they reported to have discovered a most remarkable phenomenon: the actors also possessed healing powers! Thus, they argued, a zero difference between the therapeutic effects generated by the healers and those prompted by the actors would, in fact, not indicate that spiritual healing had been ineffective. According to the consensus of our five healers, such a result was likely, and it would merely demonstrate that both types of treatment had been effective. I was baffled; if the healers were to be believed, it seemed as though we had manoeuvred ourselves into a situation where we were attempting to test an untestable hypothesis.

More discussions ensued, and eventually we came up with a new and seemingly watertight concept: we would place the healer in a cubicle adjacent to the patient, so that the patient could not see the therapist. The great appeal of this solution was that it would enable us to include a placebo group where nobody at all was present in the cubicle. With this set-up, there would be no danger of any inadvertent healing powers confounding our conclusions. But then second thoughts began to emerge: healers do not normally sit in cubicles while treating their patients. Might this abnormal situation impede their healing energy? Perhaps the one-way mirrors of the cubicle would deflect their healing energy? In this case, a negative result would again be difficult to interpret, and the healers might find reasons for declaring our trial invalid.

This point is less trivial than it may seem at first glance. When doing research, we want to make sure that any possible result can be interpreted in only one way. If two or more plausible conclusions can be drawn from it, we do not advance the existing knowledge and might even obscure the truth. We felt that it was our responsibility to design the study in such a way as to produce unambiguous results, one of the hallmarks of rigorous science.

After further discussions with our healers, we eventually reached a workable compromise: we agreed to include not two but four different treatment groups in our study. According to the final protocol, patients were allocated at random to receive one of the following four interventions:

- Healing as applied by one of our five healers in the presence of the patient;

- Placebo-healing as applied by one of our five actors pretending to be healers, in the presence of the patient;

- Healing by our healers positioned in the cubicle and hidden from the view of the patient; or, lastly,

- Placebo-healing with no human present in the cubicle.

This finally looked like a watertight study, and we were all pleased and proud to have solved these difficult methodological issues amicably. Our ideas in planning this study were indeed quite innovative: several investigators have since copied our trial design and have published results that confirm our findings. I was particularly pleased to have reached a consensual solution within a team of people coming from the most diverse backgrounds imaginable. This demonstrated, in my view, that even complex methodological issues can be tackled by individuals with no prior experience in research, provided one set of experts guides the other and real teamwork is allowed to develop.

All that was left to do now was to obtain approval from our local ethics committee and sort out a handful of logistical details; after that, the adventure of conducting this trial could begin.

At that point, I delegated the day-to-day running of the study to two of my co-workers who regularly briefed me on its progress. They worked hard to recruit patients, made sure the treatments were applied as specified in the protocol, motivated patients to show up for return visits, recorded the results and generally kept everyone happy. For the most part of a year, my team was busy running the trial.

During this time, I occasionally lent a helping hand to wheelchair-bound patients who had to navigate the stairs leading to our research laboratory. It was on one such occasion that I got an early glimpse of what the results of this study might show. Some of the patients whom I had previously encountered in wheelchairs I later observed walking the stairs. I was puzzled and asked: "Did I not see you in a wheelchair the other day?" "You certainly did, professor. The healing is doing me so much good that, for the first time in years, I can do without my wheelchair."

I was astonished. How could this be? I recall being so shocked that I needed to talk it over with Danielle at home. The nature of the trial meant that patients were receiving either healing or placebo — neither they nor I could be sure which. But such dramatic benefit was extraordinary in either of those situations. I awaited the results of our research with increasingly eager anticipation.

Finally the study ended. After the last patients had received their last healing session the randomization code was opened, the statistics were calculated and the results were summarized. What did they show? Was spiritual healing an effective form of pain control? Were we about to surprise the world of science with a sensation?

The findings demonstrated considerable pain reductions in all four groups but no significant difference between them. If anything, the placebo groups had experienced a little more pain relief than the patients receiving real spiritual healing. In other words, the effects patients had experienced during and after the healing sessions were due to a placebo response. Our results demonstrated how impressive this response could be—so effective, in fact, that some patients were able to abandon their wheelchairs entirely. This extraordinary response had occurred in a few patients from all four groups, and the average pain scores did therefore not differ between them. Our conclusion in the final paper was clear: "...*a specific effect of face-to-face or distant healing on chronic pain could not be demonstrated...*"

Once we presented the results to our five healers and other interested parties, lively and at times emotional discussions ensued. Some people argued that our findings proved how very useful healing truly was: after all, many patients had experienced significant pain reduction. Therefore, they urged us *not* to publish the findings, particularly not with the conclusions we proposed to draw. If we went ahead with our plan to report that spiritual healing relied entirely on a placebo effect, we would inevitably deprive thousands of patients of the obvious remarkable and clinically important benefit healing had to offer.

My opinion, and fortunately that of the rest of my team, was, however, quite different: yes, we had demonstrated the amazing power of the placebo effect, but we had also shown that spiritual healing was nothing more than a placebo. It was important that health care professionals and patients knew the truth. Deliberately refraining from revealing our results would make a mockery of our research. The conclusions of our study were very clear; however, the implications and recommendations that would follow from them were a different matter. The practical implications of our results depended on a range of factors that were not directly related to our study. For instance, an important next step would now be that our trial needed to be replicated by an independent team of researchers. Not to publish our results at all would prevent this crucial process and was therefore not an option. Unpublished science, I had always been taught, is no science.

This debate also had serious ethical implications. Contrary to my critics' assertions, I had no desire whatever to prevent patients from benefitting from alternative therapies. I did, however, feel duty bound to make sure that, in future, patients would receive the best available treatment—and the best available treatment is not merely a placebo, but a therapy that generates beneficial effects in addition to those induced by a placebo response.

Any effective treatment—effective beyond placebo that is—will generate a specific effect *plus* a placebo effect, provided that clinicians administer it with sufficient time, dedication, compassion and empathy. These non-specific effects, as experts often call them, are essential elements in health care and, most likely, they were the reason why the patients in our spiritual healing study had experienced less pain. Yet while non-specific effects are clearly useful, they can never be a sufficient reason for deliberately using placebos in place of established treatments. Clinicians who only apply placebos—when there is an effective therapy available—are in effect cheating their patients out of something that is often essential in bringing about a return to good health.

Others criticized our research because they felt that the reductionist approach of a randomized clinical trial is intrinsically incompatible with alternative medicine. Alternative medicine, they felt, is far too holistic, subtle and individual to be assessed by the standard scientific methodology. Again, I disagreed. A randomized clinical trial is the best research tool for providing reliable estimates of the effectiveness of a therapeutic intervention. Our lengthy discussions with the five healers had clearly demonstrated this to be true. The healers had originally wanted us to evaluate the effect of their treatment by measuring the pain of their patients before and after their therapy and subsequently calculating the difference between the two measurements. This would have certainly been much easier to do. We would not have needed to think about what might be an adequate placebo, and we would not have required any control groups, which in turn would have drastically reduced the number of patients we needed to recruit for our trial. Yet this approach would have generated a misleading impression: by disregarding any consideration of the placebo response, it would have wrongly implied that the spiritual healing itself was the sole effective agent in alleviating pain. Remarkably, our healers were able to resolve the methodological issues with us and eventually agree on a study design that would provide a fair and conclusive answer to the research question we had decided to tackle.

They were able to comprehend that all symptoms, particularly pain, can improve over time, often even without therapy. Such symptoms can also respond to the patient's own expectations, or to a multitude of other circumstances. The crucial point about a clinical trial is that it is a test that should give a reliable result about the value of the treatment *per se*. A properly planned, rigorously conducted and adequately analysed clinical trial can not only determine whether the observed outcome was caused by the therapy rather than by non-specific effects, but it can also avoid the problem of false positive or false negative findings.

Let me explain:

A false positive finding suggests that a treatment or intervention was effective when in fact it was not. Conversely, a false negative finding is a result that erroneously suggests that a treatment does *not* work when, in fact, it is effective.

In our spiritual healing study, a false negative result could have occurred for a range of reasons. If, for instance, the group of patients which we recruited had been too small, the statistical tests might have failed to show a significant difference in pain reduction between the groups despite there really being one. Therefore we had to make sure to include a sufficiently large number of patients. But there were many other potential pitfalls as well: if, for example, we had only asked one healer to perform the treatment, this person might have been useless at his job and we might have ended up inadvertently testing the skills of that particular healer rather than testing the effectiveness of the treatment overall. We thus recruited five healers of good reputation within their profession.

If we had chosen patients with a medical condition that the healers had not been confident that they could treat effectively, a negative result would have been a foregone conclusion, and our study would have been little more than a shabby debunking job. For instance, no healer I know claims to treat hair loss. It would therefore have been easy to find 100 bald men and demonstrate how utterly ineffective healers are at re-growing hair. We had to be certain to choose a condition that, in the opinion and experience of the healers, was likely to respond optimally to their therapy. Similarly, if we had used an insensitive method of measuring pain, we might have missed an effect that was, in fact, present. Luckily, we were able to choose from several properly validated means of quantifying pain.

A false positive finding, by contrast, is a result that erroneously suggests that a treatment *does* work when, in fact, it is not effective. This can happen all too easily in poorly designed clinical trials, particularly if they are open to bias. For instance, if we had allowed the healers or the patients to decide who received healing and who got the placebo, expectation of an effect would most likely have created a false positive impression. Therefore, it was important to allocate patients by chance, i.e. through a process of randomization, rather than by individual choice. A similar error might have arisen if the patient or the researcher evaluating the results had known which patient belonged to which treatment group. Thus we had to "blind" both parties to the treatment allocation. Not only that, but we also had to determine how successful our attempt to blind our patients had been. Blinding, in turn, was only possible once we had developed a placebo treatment that, to the patients, was indistinguishable from the actual healing intervention.

In the end, we had collaboratively designed what is technically called a randomized, placebo-controlled, double blind trial with four parallel groups — and, remarkably, we had done so not because the methodologists had dictated this type of study but because, after many long discussions and debates, we had arrived at a consensus amongst all parties concerned.

The randomized, placebo-controlled, double blind trial is the design that seems to engender great scepticism and wariness among many proponents of alternative medicine. Had we made a point of insisting from the outset that we were planning to conduct such a study, our healers might have flatly declined to participate. Instead, we debated and re-debated all the issues with them and let them find for themselves the most appropriate, most logical common sense solutions to the problems that emerged while designing the study. All the features of such a study serve the purpose of rendering the results reliable and of making as sure as possible that they are not influenced by bias, and can thus be interpreted clearly and unambiguously. In other words, these features are important for maximizing the likelihood that the results of a trial will actually test whether the observed effect is caused only by the treatment or by some other factors out of our control.

Without randomization, blinding and placebo controls, nobody could have been sure what the cause of the observed effect had truly been. If we had noticed a difference in pain reduction between the four groups of patients, and if the safeguards of randomization and double-blinding, etc. had not been in place, it would have been entirely reasonable to conclude that an observed effect might have been due to the expectation of the patient, or to the encouragement of the healer, or to other phenomena not directly related to the spiritual healing intervention itself. The question of cause and effect — that is, whether the outcome is directly and entirely due to the intervention — can only be determined if a clinical trial is designed to exclude possible causes other than the treatment itself.

Of course, clinical trials are not infallible. Of course, they can be flawed, and, of course, they can produce misleading results or lead to inaccurate conclusions. I have not yet met anyone in any branch of health care who would claim otherwise. The point, though, is that, until we have a better tool for testing the effectiveness of therapeutic interventions, clinical trials are without a shadow of a doubt the best tool we have — or, to borrow a famous aphorism, clinical trials are the worst research tool for determining therapeutic effectiveness of medical treatments, except for all other tools we presently have at our disposal.

Because clinical trials can never be 100 per cent fool proof, it is advisable not to rely on just one single trial when issuing general recommendations. In fact, whenever possible, it is by far better to make sure that, for therapeutic decisions, *all* the available studies, particularly those which are of high quality, are taken into consideration—and this requires what is termed a "systematic review".

A systematic review is an exhaustive examination and discussion of all the available published research that has been carried out on a given topic. Conducting a systematic review necessitates digging out all the studies that have ever been conducted on the given subject, often a tedious and time-consuming exercise requiring a considerable amount of skilled detective work. This task must be performed diligently because it is the only sure way to avoid cherry picking—that is, selecting those studies that, for whatever reason, we happen to like while ignoring those that don't support our position or the hypothesis we're developing. Next, we must critically assess the quality of the trials that we have identified; that is to say, we must evaluate the soundness of their results and conclusions and weigh the possibility of their having produced a biased, misleading, false negative or false positive result. Finally, we summarize what the best trials tell us. This process of summarizing the findings of multiple studies can sometimes require a statistical approach, in which case we are dealing with what experts call a "meta-analysis".

Systematic reviews are much more reliable than single trials because, by virtue of the sheer number of different studies from different investigators they involve, they minimize the play of chance as well as the influence of bias. They are therefore generally accepted to be the most trustworthy source of evidence in health care. This is one important reason why, over the years, our research in Exeter focused more and more on this type of research.

In the case of spiritual healing, we conducted a systematic review that we later updated when new evidence had become available. Initially, the evidence seemed mixed and at times contradictory but, once our trial design had been adopted by other investigators and further rigorous studies had emerged, the totality of the reliable clinical trials generated a fairly clear picture which confirmed the findings of our study: "...*the evidence [is] against the notion that distant healing is more than a placebo.*"

Our healing study was a typical example of the difficulties in designing research in alternative medicine but, at the same time, it also showed that, formidable though they were, the obstacles in the way of high quality trials can be overcome. This study was one of the first that my Exeter team conducted. Over the years, we published around 40 more clinical trials — always trying to incorporate the views and expertise of the therapists — and well over 300 systematic reviews.

With some alternative therapies, designing clinical trials can be fairly straightforward. For instance, when testing treatments that are taken by mouth, we usually do not encounter significant obstacles in controlling for placebo effects. It is relatively easy to "blind" patients and their physicians, and to give placebos to those allocated to the control group. Thus our trials of a weight loss aid, of homeopathic arnica, of Bach Flower Remedies, of a garlic supplement or of a Ginkgo biloba supplement all gave us relatively few problems in that respect.

In other areas of alternative medicine, though, things can be much trickier. We often had to develop innovative concepts and new ideas to solve the methodological problems we encountered. What, for instance, might constitute an adequate placebo for a trial testing the effectiveness of acupuncture? This question had intrigued the field of acupuncture research for quite some time. Several investigators had used needling at non-acupuncture points; others had opted to insert needles only superficially into the skin; others still had used acupuncture points that, by general consensus, were not indicated for the condition in question. Whenever such trials had not generated the desired positive result, acupuncturists had argued that the placebo intervention was not entirely inert, and that therefore the negative result was not valid. Such studies, they were convinced, showed no difference between acupuncture and sham-acupuncture simply because both interventions were effective. For them, paradoxically, each such negative finding was merely a confirmation of the effectiveness, and not of the ineffectiveness, of acupuncture. Due to such arguments, very little progress was being made in answering the crucial question: is the benefit which many patients experience after acupuncture caused by the treatment *per se*, or is it the result of a range of non-specific effects such as, for instance, the expectations of the practitioner, the patient or both?

To end this frustratingly fruitless dispute, we started a project to develop an acupuncture needle that would only appear to penetrate the skin while, in fact, it retracted into itself like a stage dagger, thus fooling the patient into believing that he was receiving real treatment while in fact he was not. After our PhD student had formally validated this method, we conducted a clinical trial with more than 100 patients who had suffered a stroke. Previous studies had found encouraging results suggesting that such patients would regain their bodily functions faster and more completely if they received acupuncture as an add-on to conventional rehabilitative therapy. If true, this would be an important finding: many of us suffer from a stroke during our later years. For most patients this is a devastating event from which recovery is often slow and incomplete. Any treatment that would improve this distressing situation would be more than welcome. Sadly, using our placebo needle, we found that the sham-acupuncture group in our trial recovered just as fast and as well as the patients who had received real acupuncture. We had little choice but to conclude that acupuncture is not superior to sham treatment, which must have been disappointing to enthusiasts of this treatment.

We had thus generated what is often called a "negative" result, i.e. a finding that failed to show that the tested intervention worked as claimed by its proponents. But the word "negative", in colloquial parlance at least, has pejorative connotations. Why is it considered "'negative" if medical experts and stroke patients discover that a treatment, in this case acupuncture, does not speed up recovery from a stroke? As I see it, far from being negative, it is actually the opposite, enabling everyone concerned to direct limited health resources towards treatments which demonstrably work instead of wasting money and time on those that don't. Seen from this perspective, the notion of such a result being inherently negative is misleading. The term "negative" should perhaps be reserved for a clinical trial that proves to be untrue and misleads people, thus hindering progress.

Clinical trials have always been my favourite research tool. In alternative medicine, however, they tend to be both methodologically challenging and extremely expensive to conduct. Grants for medical research are always highly competitive but the shortage of funding is particularly marked in alternative medicine research. Eventually a lack of funds led to our having to reconsider clinical trials as our primary research approach. Whenever possible we did, of course, continue with clinical trials, but now we began honing our expertise in conducting systematic reviews, eventually publishing more than 300 such projects. This figure dwarfs the number of our clinical trials, and today we are internationally best known not for the 40 clinical trials but for the abundance of our systematic reviews.

***

Evaluating the effectiveness of alternative treatments is, of course, important—but not as important, in my view, as the investigation of their safety. I had already made this point unmistakably clear in the mission statement and I was determined to adhere to it.

Proponents of alternative medicine were often *irritated* by what they saw as unnecessary and potentially damaging lines of enquiry. They were quick to point out that many more patients are being harmed on a daily basis by mainstream pharmaceuticals than by alternative treatments. As a general rule, this is probably true, and I certainly never challenged the veracity of this assertion. What I vehemently disagreed with was the implication that, simply because pharmaceuticals often have serious side effects, the risks of alternative medicine should be spared scrutiny. This seemed to me to be a total *non sequitur*. If we do not systematically investigate alternative treatments, we cannot be sure exactly how safe they are, or indeed whether any safety issues exist. And if we fail to recognize existing problems, we cannot address them. As I see it, there is no more important issue in clinical medicine than patient safety, and for any treatment to be adopted based only on unproven assumptions is inherently unethical.

Moreover, the absolute risk of any treatment is in many ways not a useful concept for estimating the value of a therapy. Any responsible therapeutic decision needs to take into account not only the risks of a certain treatment but also its anticipated benefit. If the benefit of a given intervention is small, uncertain or non-existent, then even a relatively minor risk might tilt the risk–benefit balance into the negative. If a herbal remedy, for instance, shortens the symptoms of a common cold by a few hours but, at the same time, causes severe allergic reactions in a sizable percentage of patients, no responsible health care professional would recommend it for general use.

In this context, there was a further argument to consider, one that I had quietly hoped might get alternative practitioners more firmly on my side. If their assertions about the safety of alternative medicine were correct, my research would only confirm them. Surely, I thought, this must be an aim worth fighting for, and an argument that would get the support of the alternative medicine lobby. The logic seemed to me to be unassailable; but did it win over the alternative practitioners? The short answer, I am afraid, is no.

Over the years, I had to get used to an incessant drumbeat of hostile criticism, aggression and even personal attacks. Many people, regardless of their background, status, knowledge or expertise, felt they knew so much better than I did. This often bordered on the absurd: sometimes it seemed that a critic's conviction in pressing the point was inversely proportional to his understanding of the issues at hand. I had studied my subject in depth, had earned two higher degrees, had years of clinical experience, hundreds of publications and even a dozen scientific awards to my name, yet none of this prevented others who had no qualifications, expertise or experience whatsoever from forcefully and often insultingly expressing their ill-informed opinions about research in general or my work in particular. A constant stream of letters, telephone calls and emails reminded me in no uncertain terms that I was an impostor, unqualified, wilfully wrong, misguided, stupid, corrupt and so on. At meetings with proponents or practitioners of alternative medicine, I was frequently left in no doubt that many people vehemently disagreed with me, and more than once the level of aggression became such that I felt concerned about my safety.

This was an entirely new experience for me, I have to admit, and something of a culture shock. In Vienna, I had been *Herr Professor*, someone whom nobody would dream of criticizing, at least not openly. On my becoming the Professor of Complementary Medicine at the University of Exeter, however, the climate had drastically changed. Now every Tom, Dick and Harry seemed to want to correct my concepts, reinterpret my results or question my background, attitude, integrity or intellect.

Initially, I thought this tsunami of criticism was quite refreshing in a perverse sort of way, coming as it did as an agreeable contrast to the stuffy atmosphere of Vienna. Since I was advocating critical thinking, there was, of course, no reason why I should be exempt from criticism myself. Indeed, in the beginning I was often able to see the funny side of it: for instance, getting vehemently attacked by homeopaths for not having any formal qualifications in homeopathy is hilarious considering that, in the UK (and in many other countries), no qualifications whatever are required to practise or research homeopathy.

For the first 10 years or so of my tenure at Exeter, I did my best to avoid open confrontation no matter how exasperated I was with all the mud-slinging. Later, though, when the criticism had turned into constant meddling and overt aggression, threats, and official complaints to my university peers, I slowly began to tire of it. To be taken seriously, criticism requires a basis in logic and fact; if it has neither, it does not deserve the title.

Eventually I began to stand up to the barrage, politely explaining the facts and the science behind them. I did this in publications, in lectures, in discussions, in newspapers, on the radio, on television and on the internet. And I did this not once or twice; I did it over and over again, dozens if not hundreds of times. Inevitably, though, about 15 years into my Exeter job, my patience wore thin and I began to feel that, at least on some occasions, it was probably best to show more determination or even teeth. I became more outspoken and often did not mince my words, but that only seemed to provoke more vitriolic attacks.

Slowly but surely I became resigned to the fact that, for some alternative medicine zealots, no amount of explanation would ever suffice. To them, alternative medicine seemed to have mutated into a religion, a cult whose central creed must be defended at all costs against the infidel.

If a researcher takes his job of critically evaluating alternative medicine really seriously, it is highly likely that he will be perceived as the great Satan by those who make their living from it. Conversely, if someone conducting research into alternative medicine is liked by the majority of alternative practitioners, he is almost certainly not doing his job correctly. Intriguingly, this concept is today known as "Ernst's Law".

***

In the late 1990s we carried out what was then the largest prospective study ever to investigate the safety of an alternative therapy. We persuaded 78 acupuncturists across the UK to report all adverse effects that occurred in a total of about 32,000 acupuncture sessions. While adverse effect surveillance is, of course, mandatorily and routinely performed in conventional medicine, there is no such oversight or monitoring in the world of alternative medicine; in fact, our project was a complete novelty in alternative medicine. Even though it was merely a research project and not an attempt to implement compulsory safety monitoring into everyday acupuncture practice (a task that even today has not been realized), it was nevertheless greeted with fierce resistance by the UK acupuncture establishment, and we had a major struggle keeping enough acupuncturists on board to see this project through to its end.

The results of our study, for the first time in the history of acupuncture, demonstrated beyond reasonable doubt that acupuncture, as practised in the UK by our study participants, was a relatively safe treatment. Only about 10 per cent of the patients enrolled in the study experienced adverse effects, and the nature of these problems was mostly mild. Several years later, I was involved in an even larger German study which confirmed that, in Germany, the safety profile of acupuncture is very similar to that in the UK. Today, we globally have data from several hundred thousand patients and, essentially, the message is still the same: acupuncture, as practised by Western-trained and experienced acupuncturists, causes mild adverse effects in approximately 10 per cent of patients, and serious complications are very rare.

The world of acupuncture should have been delighted. Not only had we completed a safety study that arguably should long since have been done by acupuncturists themselves, but we had also generated a reassuring bottom line. Yet most acupuncturists seemed to think that our project had been a waste of time: in their view, it only had alerted people to the fact that acupuncture was not entirely free of side effects.

Other investigations by our team and other researchers had shown that acupuncture could, in fact, occasionally cause very severe harm. These complications were caused mostly through needles introducing infection such as HIV or hepatitis B or C into the body, or injuring a vital organ (most frequently the lungs). Such complications could result in severe health problems, even deaths. So the somewhat confusing message was that acupuncture is relatively safe, but sometimes it can cause serious problems. The most likely explanation for this apparent

contradiction is that the acupuncturists volunteering to participate in our prospective studies were mostly British and German
doctors who were, of course, generally well-trained. To put it
bluntly, they had learnt where the lungs are located within the
body, and what the sterility of a needle involves; therefore they
were not prone to puncturing a lung or infecting their patients
with hepatitis. On the other hand, traditional acupuncturists,
particularly those in Asian countries, were often completely
devoid of any medical training or education. The conclusion to
be drawn from this insight is clear and, I think, important: the
safety of acupuncture depends on who administers the treatment and where the treatment is given. The average acupuncturist in rural China, for instance, might be less well edu-
cated and trained than his UK or US counterpart, and might
therefore be more likely to use non-sterile needles or
inadvertently puncture an internal organ. In other words, when
considering the safety of an alternative treatment modality, we
need to think not just of the therapy itself but also of the therapist, the setting and the wider context in which the treatment is
administered.

The lessons from this line of research might seem obvious
but they also are important: some alternative therapies are
relatively safe; however, the same may not always be true for
the practitioners who administer them. The systematic, careful
and critical evaluation of the risks and the benefits of any
treatment is neither unnecessarily alarmist nor of purely
theoretical, academic interest. Far from it: it is prudent and
necessary to establish exactly what risks might be involved,
especially in a setting where there is no standardization of
practitioner training and no regulatory oversight of the treatment. Far from being a vendetta motivated by animus against
alternative medicine, investigating the risks of alternative
therapies constitutes valuable research aimed at ensuring consumer safety.

As a team, we were proud to have constructively contributed to showing that acupuncture, as practised by UK doctors,
does not significantly harm patients. This, I felt, represented an

important step towards achieving exactly what my chair was created for—namely, to encourage the assimilation of appropriate treatments into mainstream clinical routine, in line with the dictum that there is no such thing as alternative medicine; there are just treatments that work, and those that don't. Those that work will find their way into the standard armamentarium of medicine, while those that don't are destined to remain in the realm of quackery.

Some alternative treatments seem intrinsically much more likely to cause serious harm than acupuncture. Spinal manipulation as practised by chiropractors, for instance, turned out to be a much more hazardous therapy. Data published by chiropractors had shown conclusively that about every second patient consulting a chiropractor would experience mild to moderate adverse effects, such as an increase in pain lasting normally 1–3 days. Chiropractors insisted that such reactions were a necessary first step on the path to getting better. But was this really true? The adverse effects could be strong enough to seriously interfere with the quality of life of the patient, and it seemed entirely legitimate—even necessary—to investigate whether these risks might outweigh any possible benefit of spinal manipulation.

Imagine an equivalent scenario in the arena of drug therapy: a medication of doubtful effectiveness causing mild to moderate adverse effects for two or three days in every second patient. Would we recommend such a drug? With an adverse event profile like this, it would surely be quickly withdrawn from the market, or at the very least be compelled to carry a prominent warning to prescribers and patients alike.

In addition to these relatively minor, transient problems, hundreds of very serious complications have, over the years, been documented following chiropractic spinal manipulation. The most serious problems involved damage to arteries that supply the brain. Such damage is technically called an "arterial dissection" and can result in a stroke or even death. The explanation for these disasters is quite straightforward: extreme rotation and extension of the neck may overstretch an artery running alongside the upper spine, causing the wall of the blood vessel to rupture, resulting in a stroke.

Whenever I plucked up the courage to publish on this important subject, the chiropractic fraternity, not just in the UK but also across the globe, reacted with fury. Instead of engaging in a scientific debate, they filed complaints with my peers and tried to silence me in every way they could think of. Instead of looking at the evidence impartially, they flatly denied that neck manipulation might cause a stroke. Instead of conducting proper research to fill in the existing knowledge gaps, they ran *ad hominem* attacks against me and claimed my research was flawed. Instead of recognizing that I was merely doing what a responsible scientist in my position had to do, they claimed I was waging a war against the chiropractic profession.

Alternative practitioners in general remained deeply sceptical that research into the risks and safety of alternative medicine was a crucially important contribution to the evidence. Instead they argued that my research focus on risks amounted to an obsessive personal crusade against alternative medicine; that my conclusions were deliberately alarmist; that I was simply trying to deflect attention away from the real dangers, which were to be found exclusively among the conventional drugs of mainstream medicine; that my research was in any case flawed; that I had an axe to grind; or that I was in the pocket of Big Pharma. When our research indicated quite clearly that the reported risks were only the tip of a much bigger iceberg, alternative medicine extremists regularly redoubled their attacks, on occasion becoming openly threatening.

Things went from bad to worse when I started to investigate what I called the indirect risks of alternative medicine. Even if one particular alternative therapy was entirely devoid of risk, I argued, we still have to consider its indirect risks, by far the most important of which is the possibility that a patient will avoid an effective mainstream treatment in favour of an ineffective alternative option.

The point here is essentially very simple: even the most ostensibly harmless intervention becomes positively life-threatening if it is employed instead of an effective therapy for a serious illness. The very term "alternative medicine" illustrates this potential danger well, implying, as it does, that there is a fundamental equivalence, an interchangeableness, between standard and unconventional approaches. The extent of such substitution is, of course, difficult to investigate and reliable information is therefore scarce—with one important exception: the attitude of some alternative practitioners towards vaccination.

When Hahnemann developed homeopathy about 200 years ago, he was adamant that it should be used as an alternative to and a replacement for conventional medicine. He even went so far as to decry as "traitors" those practitioners who used homeopathy alongside mainstream treatment. In Hahnemann's time this attitude might have made sense to some degree— many conventional therapies at that period were not just ineffective but actually more dangerous than the diseases they sought to cure. Today, this is no longer the case, and most homeopaths therefore use their remedies as a complement rather than an alternative to mainstream medicine—most, but by no means all. We only need to go on the internet to find innumerable statements claiming homeopathy to be effective for every serious and treatable condition imaginable—anything from AIDS to cancer, tuberculosis or cholera. Whenever a patient is persuaded by such statements and opts to employ homeopathy instead of effective interventions, serious harm is almost unavoidable.

In 1995, I raised for the first time the concern that some UK homeopaths were advising parents against immunizing their children, claiming that their homeopathic "nosodes" are better and safer. At the time, we had published a small survey of homeopaths listed in the Exeter *Yellow Pages*, demonstrating that none of the non-medically qualified homeopaths reco-mmended immunizations. Such results were interesting but not necessarily generalizable to the wider national population because our study was far too small to draw conclusions regarding the extent of anti-vaccination sentiment across the

UK. Nevertheless, we published our findings prominently in the hope that it would trigger some discussion and perhaps even spur the country's non-medical homeopaths to reconsider their stance on the issue of vaccination.

In 2002, at the time of the MMR (measles, mumps and rubella vaccine) scare promoted by Andrew Wakefield's now discredited "research", we decided to broaden our initial pilot study to the national level. In order to accomplish this, we had obtained the email addresses of a sizable number of UK chiropractors and homeopaths, and sent a request to these practitioners. In it, a fictional mother, concerned about the conflicting press reports regarding the safety of the MMR vaccine, asked for advice on MMR vaccination for her one-year-old child. After the replies had come in, we wrote to each respondent again and explained that the query had not been genuine but was, in fact, part of a research project. At the same time, we offered all participants the chance to withdraw their answers. The study had, of course, been approved in advance by our local ethics committee, and debriefing the respondents in this way was part of the approved protocol.

In total, we managed to contact 168 homeopaths, of whom 72 per cent responded, and 26 per cent withdrew their answers after the debriefing. We also contacted 63 chiropractors, of whom 44 per cent responded initially and 27 per cent later withdrew their responses. Our analyses showed that very few homeopaths and only a quarter of the chiropractors would advise their patients in favour of the MMR vaccination. Almost half of the homeopaths and nearly a fifth of the chiropractors would recommend against immunizing.

What happened next is amazing and perhaps even unprecedented in the recent history of medical research. This seemingly innocent and insignificant research project almost cost me my job. After receiving the debriefing email, several homeopaths complained to my university peers and to our ethics committee, claiming the research was unethical because it had been conducted on non-consenting human research subjects (the homeopaths and chiropractors) who had been misled about the nature of the enquiry. In view of these complaints, our ethics committee got cold feet and took the most remarkable step of withdrawing their previous approval; not only that, they forbade us to use the results in any way.

However, at this stage of the project I had already submitted our findings as a short report for publication in the *British Medical Journal*, and I flatly refused to comply with those ridiculous demands. The article was thus published only days after this storm had started blowing.

My Exeter peers were not amused by my disobedience, decided to conduct an official investigation and ordered me to attend several interrogatory sessions. For several weeks, I thought they might find me guilty of conducting unethical research and condemn my actions which, in the worst-case scenario, could have meant disciplinary action against me. Even the mildest reprimand would have been devastating to the credibility of my research team as a whole. The homeopaths who had filed the complaint were only waiting to use such news to discredit me once and for all. Fortunately, after several highly unpleasant exchanges, I managed to convince my peers that, considering the lively public and medical debate about the risks or benefits of the MMR vaccination, a swift publication of these findings had been in the public's best interest. Eventually, it was decided that no disciplinary action, not even a reprimand, was called for.

I felt strongly then—and I still do today—that our research was not in the least unethical. In order to discover the extent and the effects of irresponsible behaviour, researchers, like police, sometimes have no choice but to conduct undercover investigations of this nature; and, whenever necessary, I continued doing so.

In a similar project, I collaborated with a London-based journalist who, pretending to be a cancer patient, visited five practitioners who offered alternative cancer cures. He personally made appointments, supplied all the necessary details and asked for advice regarding treatment of his highly treatable, and curable, form of lymphatic cancer. In the course of these five consultations, he received recommendations for a myriad unproven treatments. Had he followed the advice of these charlatans, some of whom were medical doctors, he would almost certainly have lost his life — not to mention being relieved of at least £26,000 on the way out. Studies of this nature may seem unfair and threatening to the practitioners concerned, but they are nevertheless immensely important from the perspective of public health; in fact, they can save lives.

Without a doubt, many patients choose to follow advice from irresponsible promoters of alternative medicine and forsake standard medical care entirely. Others may start by consulting alternative practitioners, and only much later, after their disease has failed to respond to quack remedies, seek proper medical care. Avoidance or delays of this kind can also be fatal, allowing a serious disease to progress beyond the point of no return.

Years after our undercover investigation into alternative practitioners' attitudes towards immunization, my friend Simon Singh repeated a similar, but much more public, sting. He recruited a volunteer to consult several homeopaths requesting their advice regarding malaria protection. The results indicated that most homeopaths would not recommend effective preventive measures but instead advised patients to use "homeopathic immunization" for which there is not a shred of evidence. His investigation was subsequently replicated twice by the television BBC *Newsnight* programme, with essentially the same results.

The inability of alternative practitioners to learn from mistakes is a phenomenon that never ceases to astound and worry me; it implies that in ten years from now homeopaths and other dogmatists might still be endangering public health with the same scientifically unsound and unproven notions that have been their proud and unwavering mainstay for 200 years. And quite probably, when they are caught with egg on their faces, they will still pretend to be right and turn their fury on the researchers who exposed them.

All too often, the public is hoodwinked into believing that everything "natural" must also be safe. This familiar marketing strategy of alternative medicine may be good for business but it is most certainly very bad for public health. Similarly, consumers are led to believe that, whether or not they actually do good, alternative practitioners cannot do much harm. Even mainstream healthcare professionals who do not necessarily accept every nonsensical claim made by alternative medicine enthusiasts tend to trivialize the issue by saying these therapists might be a bit odd but are essentially harmless.

The indisputable fact, however, is that recommendations to forgo effective mainstream medical treatments in favour of bogus cures and quackery does cost lives — not just occasionally but regularly. It is obvious why this message is not popular with those who promote alternative medicine and earn a comfortable living from it. To me, however, it is equally clear that this message needs to be told and re-told, over and over again, in order to minimize the harm that charlatans inflict on the unsuspecting and often all too trusting public.

Over the years, our team conducted research into most aspects of alternative medicine. While our principal focus had always been the safety and effectiveness of alternative therapies, we also tackled a range of other topics in this area: for instance, we investigated the reasons why consumers and patients elect to use alternative medicine; we researched how many patients are tempted to go down this route; we asked conventional practitioners about their attitude towards and knowledge of alternative medicine. As the unit grew, so did our output of published articles, books and lectures. Our reputation attracted many foreign researchers who travelled to Exeter to join the team for a few months or years. This broadened our perspective and led to a multitude of international collaborations. In turn, this activity further increased our productivity and strengthened our international position as a centre of excellence.

At least two independent assessments identified my unit as the most productive alternative medicine research team in the world. Later, some particularly mendacious commentators would claim that the sheer number of our published papers—today they amount to well over 1000—was in itself proof of fraudulent activity. It goes without saying that this is not true. The team was highly motivated; we enjoyed our work, as a unit, and we were both very industrious and highly successful. That such success attracts envy is perhaps understandable. That it also attracts defamation is, I think, an inevitable result of the fact that many of our findings challenged many of the treasured beliefs of those for whom alternative medicine functions more as a religion than as method of health care.

Chapter 6

Wonderland

It has been claimed by some members of the lunatic fringe of alternative medicine that I took up the Laing Chair at Exeter with the specific agenda of debunking alternative medicine. This is certainly not true; if anything, I was predisposed to look kindly on it. After all, I had grown up and done my medical training in Germany where the use of alternative therapies in a supportive role alongside standard medical care was considered routine and unremarkable. As a clinician, I had *seen* positive results from alternative therapies. If I came to Exeter with any preconceived ideas at all, they were of a generally favourable kind. I was sure that, if we applied the rules of science to the study of alternative medicine, we would find plenty of encouraging evidence.

As if to prove this point, the managing director of a major UK homeopathic pharmacy wrote a comment on my blog in April 2014: *"…I met you once in Exeter in the 90s when exploring a possible clinical study. I found you most encouraging and openly enthusiastic about homeopathy. I would go so far as to say I was inspired to go further in homeopathy thanks to you but now you want to close down something which in my experience does so much good in the world. What went wrong?"*

The answer to this question is fairly simple: nothing went wrong, but the evidence demonstrated more and more indisputably that most alternative therapies are not nearly as effective as enthusiasts tried to make us believe. As my research progressed and as I acquired deeper knowledge of the field, I began to view alternative medicine in a more critical light. The more data we amassed, the more we had to realize how unsubstantiated were many of the claims in support of many of these treatments. As the scientific evidence mounted, I could not help seeing what was right before my eyes. In truth, the more time I spent immersed in the world of alternative medicine, the more disillusioned I became realizing how very few of these approaches had any real therapeutic potential.

But it was not the evidence alone that brought about this gradual shift of attitude. Two further, bizarre features of the alternative medicine scene significantly contributed to this development: the strange activities of other researchers working in my field, and the many fallacious arguments commonly used by the general public to promote outright quackery.

Through my own research, our annual scientific conference at Exeter, our journal *FACT* (*Focus on Alternative and Complementary Medicine*) and through the many lectures I was giving across the globe, I got to know most researchers in alternative medicine and befriended some of them. Scrutinizing the attitudes and publications of these investigators carefully, I realized how few of them had any real intention to ever seriously question their assumptions or truly test their concepts. With a degree of simplification and little exaggeration, I could categorize my fellow investigators in two different groups:

- The researcher who avoided testing a hypothesis at all costs because this might generate a negative result which, in turn, would upset someone of influence. He would typically conduct survey after survey or interview studies or focus group research or other qualitative research. His results might show that a sizable proportion of the general public used this or that alternative therapy, that users of alternative medicine are generally very satisfied with it, that they use it for this or that ailment, that they have certain expectation, or that they happily pay out of their own pockets for it, etc. Sure, this sort of research had very little potential to upset anyone, but it also had virtually no consequences. It certainly would not improve health care or answer any of the burning questions that needed answering.

- The researcher who was blindly in love with his pet therapy might conduct clinical trials which seemingly were testing hypotheses, not least because he realized that approach was the most likely to convince the sceptics. On closer inspection, however, one would notice that these tests were set up or analysed in such a way that a positive result was pre-programmed. These pseudoscientists, as I began to call them, were on a mission and they were therefore using science as a tool not for testing but for confirming their quasi-religious beliefs. How else could 100% of a researcher's studies of an utterly implausible treatment produce positive results? How else could it be that none of his findings were ever independently replicated? How else could our research show three times in a row that the major journals of alternative medicine were publishing practically no negative findings?

Research of this nature was either irrelevant for producing real progress, or it was even preventing it. To realize how very few investigators were actually willing or able to conduct rigorous research, with an appropriate dose of critical thinking that would have enabled them to challenge their own beliefs, felt like having landed on a different planet.

The second bizarre feature of this Wonderland was the ideological fervour that permeated so much of the public discourse on alternative medicine. The need to regularly defend my research against a constant barrage of criticism would not have been so wearying had the substance of the arguments been less fallacious. A great many of the criticisms levelled with such catechistic conviction by proponents of alternative medicine were quite simply based on flawed logic. Far too many of the arguments used to defend alternative medicine represented nothing less than the flight from reason into the absurd.

In the endless discussions about the virtues of alternative medicine, I began to feel like a fish out of water. I was a physician and a clinical researcher, not a public relations specialist. Yet it became increasingly difficult for me to ignore the sloppy or irrational thinking and sophistry which more than once reminded me of Voltaire's *bon mot* that people who tolerate absurdities might also commit atrocities.

Alternative medicine had begun its remarkable ascent in a general climate of unreason. Incrementally, over the past two decades, we have seen the emergence of a culture that is curiously indifferent to the concept of truth. There is not one truth now, but many—all of them interchangeable, all of them of equal weight, and all deserving of equal consideration. In this Wonderland of relative facts, parallel truths and intellectual legerdemain, basing an argument on flawed reasoning does not automatically disqualify or even devalue it. To the contrary: logical fallacies are tolerated—indeed, often celebrated—as manifestations of a much-needed diversity.

Proponents of alternative medicine thrive in this kind of cultural environment since they tend to rely heavily on lazy reasoning and systematic oversimplification. Take, for example, the widespread notion that, if millions use a certain therapy, it can safely be assumed that it is effective—a prime example of what is known in logic as the "*ad populum*" fallacy.

A belief—even mass-belief—can be wrong; a widely accepted practice, habit or tradition can still be misguided. Popularity is certainly not a reliable barometer of effectiveness. The history of medicine is littered with examples demonstrating how dangerous this fallacy can be. Bloodletting, purges, mercury cures were all, at one time or another, widely practised and believed to be effective—and yet these treatments undoubtedly killed more patients than they ever cured. If we followed the logic of proponents of alternative medicine and allowed medicine to degenerate into a popularity contest, we would automatically jeopardize all the remarkable achievements that have been made in the last 150 years.

Similarly beguiling is the widespread confusion of cause and effect, exemplified by the notion that, because event B followed event A, event B must have been caused by event A. This kind of thinking, known as the *post hoc* fallacy, is nowhere more pervasive than in alternative medicine. If we receive a therapy while we are ill and soon afterwards get better, we automatically assume that the treatment was responsible for our improvement. Tempting though this conclusion may be, it can be dangerously misleading. A whole spectrum of phenomena, ranging from the placebo effect to the self-limiting nature of the illness itself, can contribute to the recovery of ill patients. Patients do usually get better after receiving a useless or even mildly harmful remedy. To assume a cause and effect relationship based on purely temporal associations of this kind is always unreliable and certainly does not provide a sufficient basis on which to draw conclusions about the efficacy of a therapy.

When apologists for alternative medicine have to concede that their treatment is ineffective, they usually insist that this does not really matter. Even if it were a pure placebo, it would nevertheless help patients by eliciting a placebo response, and that, in and of itself, surely must be a good thing. According to this fuzzy line of reasoning, the mechanism of the effect is of secondary importance; the only thing that truly counts is to help the patient by whatever means one can.

Superficially, the assumption sounds logical enough—and compassionate, too—but it ignores several important points. The administration of placebos to ill patients can be both unethical and dangerous. For example, as discussed in the previous chapter, some forms of alternative medicine are by no means inert: they can cause serious adverse effects in their own right. Also, in order to elicit a placebo response, it is not necessary to administer a placebo. If a clinician gives his patient an effective treatment with empathy and compassion, he will generate a placebo response in addition to the response to the effective treatment he has chosen for his patient. Only giving a placebo therefore deprives the patient of the benefits of a treatment that has specific therapeutic effects in its own right. In other words, the administration of placebo therapies would simply mean cheating the patient out of something that would contribute importantly to his recovery—and this, surely, is unethical and potentially harmful.

Another false but superficially convincing argument loved by proponents of alternative medicine holds that many conventional treatments are not supported by sound evidence. They point out that, since standard medical treatments are by no means always backed up by solid proof, it must be unreasonable to insist on a solid evidence-base for alternative therapies. As they see it, this reveals an entrenched double standard and an institutionalized bias against alternative medicine.

It is unquestionably true that many conventional therapies are currently not evidence-based, but this is by no means a justification for using untested or disproven treatments under the banner of alternative medicine. This logic would be like arguing that unreliable (or unsafe) railways are acceptable because many more people get stuck in traffic jams (or die in accidents) on the roads. If we identify treatments as being unproven, we have a duty to test them; and until the results are in we should stop using them in clinical routine. This is precisely what is happening in conventional medicine. However, in alternative health care, the opposite is usually the case: here apologists try to push their treatments regardless of the evidence, arguing that, as long as their therapy is not disproven, it is fine to use it. Far from decreasing the total number of non-evidence-based therapies, this approach would dramatically increase it.

Another version of this argument alludes to the fact that one of the most frequent causes of illness is the harm caused by prescription drugs. I hear it with unfailing regularity when I lecture about the risks of alternative medicine: in comparison to the number and seriousness of adverse effects attributable to prescription drugs, those caused by alternative medicine are vanishingly small. The implication here is, of course, that researchers should just stop worrying people with their concerns about the safety of some alternative therapies.

It is undoubtedly correct that the risks of some conventional treatments are far greater than those of most alternative therapies: chemotherapy has more side effects than aromatherapy, for instance. But this platitude is entirely beside the point. The true value of a treatment is definitely not determined by its absolute risk but by the balance between risk and benefit. If a treatment is potentially life-saving, even substantial risks will be offset by the benefit to be gained. If, for instance, the aim is to cure a cancer, patients will gladly put up with all sorts of dramatic and unpleasant side effects. If, however, a therapy has no, or very little, proven benefit—and this seems to be the case with many alternative treatments—even a small risk must weigh heavily.

An all-time favourite argument of alternative medicine's more passionate adherents holds that, somehow, alternative medicine defies science or extends beyond the boundaries of science as it is currently understood. Therefore, they claim, it cannot be tested in the same way one would test a conventional treatment. Some practitioners argue that their particular therapy is holistic, individualized and complex; that it relies on subtle, unquantifiable energies, etc. These attributes, they insist, mean that it cannot be squeezed into the straightjacket of reductionist science. After all, they say, science is not the only way of knowing or finding the truth: there are many things in heaven and earth which science will never be able to explain.

It is true that science does indeed have its limitations; nobody would deny that. Yet, when it comes to testing thera-peutic claims, science provides us with a fairly comprehensive set of tools for checking their validity. Even if the hypothesis is that a particular holistic, individualized and complex form of energy healing makes patients somehow feel better, live longer or experience life more wholesomely, the hypothesis is scientifically testable. And even if, for a particular claim, no validated outcome measure exists, scientists would certainly be able to develop one. The notion of "my therapy defies scientific testing" merely discloses a lack of understanding as to what science can achieve—or, more likely, a fear of being tested and found wanting—or, even more likely, an attempt to mislead consumers.

In health care it is unwise, dangerous and arguably unethical to give "the benefit of the doubt" to under-researched therapies. In the best interest of patients, we should ideally employ only treatments that are supported by sound evidence; and this clearly means that we have to consider all interventions to be ineffective until sound data to the contrary are available. Yet many proponents of alternative medicine like to stress that the absence of evidence of an effect does not constitute evidence of the absence of an effect. In other words, just because we have no evidence on the effectiveness or safety of a particular type of alternative medicine, we cannot simply assume that it is ineffective or unsafe.

The principle is, of course, theoretically correct: we have not identified life on other planets, for instance, but we cannot be sure that no extraterrestrial life exists. However, the conclusion some enthusiasts of alternative medicine draw from this principle is fallacious. They like to argue that, until evidence emerges which proves that a treatment is ineffective, it is reasonable or in the best interest of patients to continue using the treatment in question. Intriguingly, the people using this argument are usually the quickest to decry scientists' attempts to evaluate the very methods that they espouse so passionately.

A particularly seductive idea — often one that need only be subtly implied rather than overtly stated — is that alternative medicine is intrinsically more compassionate than conventional medical care. This argument has instant resonance with a public that is all too familiar with the harried physician whose time is always limited and who often does a less than perfect job of answering questions and anticipating patients' concerns. Indeed, one of the major influences fuelling the growth of alternative medicine during recent decades has been the quest for a lengthier and more personal interaction with the caregiver.

In my experience, it is true that many alternative practitioners are full of good intentions and often manage to cultivate a friendly and empathetic therapeutic relationship with their patients which may well have useful potential in its own right. However, to extrapolate from this that alternative therapies are therefore effective or useful is little more than a self-serving delusion. There is nothing intrinsically heartless about conventional medicine, nor does alternative medicine have a uniquely gentle, caring ethos. Compassion, empathy and good patient–clinician interactions are not the exclusive purview of any particular branch of medicine. On the contrary, they are the hallmarks of any good health care, whatever its philosophical or therapeutic orientation.

Many forms of alternative medicine have a long history, and proponents use this undeniable fact to convince the public of its value. Any treatment that has passed the test of time, they say, must be effective and safe — after all, people are not stupid: why would they persist in using such treatments if they did not work or if they caused harm? Some alternative medicine enthusiasts even view the "test of time" as more relevant than any objective evaluation. Clinical trials, they insist, are of necessity artificial and relatively small-scale, while tradition is real and large-scale. A long history of use is therefore a more conclusive test than science can ever provide.

An established tradition can, of course, be a valuable indicator suggesting that a treatment is safe and effective, but it can never provide solid proof. A long history might simply mean that the origins of that particular therapy reach back to the days when the basic medical sciences such as anatomy, biochemistry and physiology were not well understood; in this case, it might merely disclose a significant weakness in its foundations.

In an attempt to promote wider acceptance of their particular alternative model, devotees often invoke the support of authority. They may, for instance, state that the UK National Health Service endorses their particular modality; or that, in China, acupuncture is supported by the government; or that respectable nationwide pharmacy chains sell their products; or that the Royal family or some other celebrities use this treatment; or that Nobel Prize winners support it, etc. These claims might well be true, but one cannot infer from them that the treatment in question must therefore be valuable. The fact that any person or institution, however well respected, praises or adopts something never constitutes proof of anything. It might merely illustrate that even well-educated people or powerful institutions can sometimes commit the silliest and most obvious of mistakes.

An entire industry has developed around the fallacious concept that, because something is natural, it cannot do any harm. Implicit in this notion is the perception that conventional medicine is somehow inherently unnatural, relying heavily on drugs that are derived from harmful synthetic chemicals. Nature, by contrast, is seen as benign, and natural remedies are therefore not just intrinsically superior but also safer.

While undoubtedly clever for marketing purposes, this argument is nevertheless false and in many instances even dangerous. By no means are all forms of alternative medicine natural or benign. For instance, there is nothing natural in sticking needles into a patient's body (as in acupuncture), or endlessly diluting and shaking a medicine (as in homeopathy), or in introducing gallons of tepid coffee to the large intestine via the rectum (as in the coffee enemas so beloved by many alternative practitioners). Moreover, nature is by no means always benevolent, as anyone who has been out at sea through heavy weather or had the misfortune to be hit by lightning knows all too well. Even "natural" plant extracts are not necessarily safe — just think of hemlock.

It is perhaps not surprising that such irrational worldviews often include a hefty component of paranoia. Conspiracy theories and persecution complexes are the preferred way of some alternative medicine zealots to explain why mainstream medicine continues to ignore their anointed approach to health care. With unfailing regularity they claim that powerful forces are at work to suppress their time-honoured wisdom about health care. The pharmaceutical industry — Big Pharma — is almost invariably implicated as the chief villain in this context. The fevered plot has it that the pharmaceutical industry is systematically sabotaging alternative medicine because it would lose substantial amounts of revenue if the true value of this or that form of alternative medicine were to become general knowledge.

During my many years of researching alternative medicine, I have never seen a scintilla of evidence to suggest this allegation to be true; nor can those who make such charges ever produce good evidence to substantiate them. In my experience, the pharmaceutical industry is barely aware of the alternative medicine industry — when it is, it usually finds ways of profiting from it, for example by marketing "natural" dietary supplements.

Next to the arch-villain Big Pharma, the medical profession comes a close second. Oncologists in particular are singled out as ruthless conspirators, single-mindedly suppressing alternative cancer "cures". So far, I have not met one oncologist who would not be delighted to have access to further effective cancer cures without caring a damn whether they originated from the field of alternative medicine or from any other source. Furthermore, if there were indeed effective natural, alternative cancer cures known to — but suppressed by — oncologists, no oncologist, nor any friend, colleague or family member of an oncologist, would ever die of cancer. Yet they are just as likely as anyone else to fall victim to this category of diseases.

We live in times where political correctness regularly drives us to look for the middle ground in areas where there simply is none. Journalists are particularly apt to kowtow to ideological orthodoxy in this way. For example, a health journalist writing an article about homeopathy might diligently present all the facts about the implausibility of the rationale on which homeopathy is based, and the lack of evidence to suggest that it has consistent, replicable value in the treatment of illness. But, obedient to the *zeitgeist* of cultural relativism, the journalist would also feel obliged to "balance" this with input from the "other side" — i.e. with quotes from a homeopath who says that science cannot know everything and his personal experience is more important than scientific data.

This would, of course, be fair enough, provided there were a reasonable "other side" whose arguments had weight and substance. If, however, the "other side" is not of equivalent substance, this insistence on balance creates the erroneous impression that there is a continuing, valid scientific debate between two equal hypotheses, while, in fact, there is complete consensus and the science has long been settled. The discussion as to whether the earth is flat or a sphere is as closed as is that concerning homeopathy. Imagine that *National Geographic* were to publish an article "balancing" existing scientific knowledge by presenting the opinions of a member of the Flat Earth Society. Who would take it seriously? Yet we regularly accept the equivalent when discussing homeopathy. In some areas of alternative medicine, the insistence on a middle ground approach is not only unreasonable but also misleading and potentially dangerous.

When the enemies of reason run out of arguments there is always the time-tested *ad hominem* fallacy to fall back on. The sole purpose of *ad hominem* attacks is to discredit one's opponent—and, in pursuit of this noble end, the *ad hominem* assailants need not trouble themselves with inconvenient little details such as ethics or truth. Instead, they can give their imagination free rein to invent whatever fanciful possibilities they need in order to lend weight to their assaults. During the 20 years I spent researching alternative medicine, I was on the receiving end of more than my fair share of such personal attacks, and one of the most insistently repeated assertions is the myth that I was being paid by Big Pharma to tarnish the reputation of alternative medicine. It goes without saying that this allegation is untrue; but how can I prove it? Perhaps the fact that my unit had to close because of lack of financial support might convince my detractors—according to their own logic, research funds from Big Pharma should have been endless.

All of these disparate smokescreens, errors, conspiracy theories, follies and fallacies are used in Wonderland as tools with one common purpose: to mislead the public such that even the most extravagant absurdities of alternative medicine appear plausible. Collectively they help foster and perpetuate a culture of unreason that is essential for the survival of alternative medicine. In essence, they constitute an attack upon rationality and a treason against progress in health care.

But undoubtedly the most useful tool of all is an influential person, a figurehead behind whom the enemies of reason can be counted on to rally obediently, a leader who can motivate and direct them in their rejection of science and the ideas of enlightenment. Different countries and different historical tides bring forth their own figureheads; in the UK the alternative medicine lobby and the forces of irrationality must surely count themselves lucky to have found their supreme champion, their unlikely Goliath, in the person of the Prince of Wales.

Chapter 7

Off With His Head!

With the wisdom of hindsight, it is clear to me now that my hope of bringing the scientific method to bear on alternative medicine was doomed from the start. Reason cannot negotiate with unreason any more than fire and water can commingle peacefully. In either case, a great deal of spitting and hissing is bound to ensue — and precious little else.

Soon after arriving in Exeter, in 1993, I learnt of the long-standing interest Prince Charles had in alternative medicine: he had asked via my Vice Chancellor for a copy of my inaugural lecture, and I remember being delighted at this request. As I never give lectures or speeches from a script, I even composed a summary specifically for him. In return, I received a polite note of thanks from one of his secretaries. This is great, I thought.

I was thrilled that someone as influential as Prince Charles would be interested in my work. What could be better than having support in such high places? Surely, there would come the time when I could meet the Prince and have an open exchange of views. I had no doubt that he would be keenly aware of the obvious necessity for rigorous research — in fact, he often enough had publicly stressed it — and would thus support my research endeavours.

How wrong can one be? Prince Charles turned out to be no supporter of my work. To the contrary: he seemed to be a staunch advocate of unreason and a formidable opponent of any attempt to bring science or critical thinking to bear on alternative medicine. What is more, subsequent events suggested to me that his intervention played a part in the closure of my unit.

Had I known more about his background I might have anticipated most of this. Because of his long-standing interest in health care, the British Medical Association (BMA) had elected Prince Charles as their president in 1982 when he was just 33 years of age. In December 1982, he gave his presidential address to the assembly. The surprise of these well-seasoned and experienced physicians must have been considerable when, instead of praising the achievements of modern health care or the BMA, the future King of England delivered a paean to alternative medicine, taking pains to point out that "the whole of the imposing edifice of modern medicine, for all its breath-taking success is, like the celebrated Tower of Pisa, slightly off balance". Alternative medicine, he went on to say, "can bring considerable relief, if not hope, to an increasing number of people".

As a direct reaction to Prince Charles's speech, the shell-shocked BMA officials obediently established a working party to look into alternative medicine. Four years later, this committee published their report. Now it was Prince Charles's turn to be knocked off kilter. The BMA had arrived at the view that alternative medicine was based on discredited philosophies and identified "no logical class of alternative therapies". The report also stated that there are "only therapies with, and without, good evidence for their efficacy". Essentially, the BMA seemed to deny alternative medicine any role whatsoever in modern health care.

As Prince Charles himself later described it, "all hell broke loose". Instead of causing him to reconsider his position, the BMA's rebuff seemed only to enforce the Prince's determination to advance the cause of alternative medicine at every opportunity. Over the years, he has done this with an increasingly anti-scientific stance, at one occasion even admitting that he felt "rather proud" of being "an enemy of the Enlightenment".

Several years after that initial dramatic and no doubt formative exchange with the BMA, Prince Charles decided to host a series of meetings at the Royal Society of Medicine in London, entitled "Talking Health". At one of these events, he declared:

"Scientific progress comes as much through deductive logic, rational debate and critical evaluation as it does through intuitive reasoning, creative play and the ability to tolerate uncertainty." Prince Charles continued expressing his hope that "a situation will develop by which the general practitioner can recommend genuine complementary therapies to treat his patients". At the time, Dr Patrick Pietroni served as the Prince's advisor on matters related to alternative medicine, and it was he who distilled the arguments to their bare essence and unnerving simplicity: "I believe we have too much and not too little research."

Ironically, it was as a direct consequence of these "Talking Health" meetings that my chair at Exeter was created. One of the people attending was Sir Maurice Laing, who argued that alternative medicine could not possibly go anywhere in the UK unless a full professorial chair were established at a British university. Later, Sir James Watt, who had chaired these meetings, took the matter up with him and asked him to fund such a chair. Sir Maurice agreed, Exeter eventually got the money, and the rest is history.

Since then, Prince Charles has continued to promote alternative medicine indefatigably, often showing himself unwilling or unable to distinguish between real health care and blatant quackery, between medicine and snake oil, or between the truth and some half-baked obsessions of his own.

In his book *Harmony: A New Way Of Looking At Our World*, Prince Charles makes the claim, for instance, that "rivers flow just as our blood flows, by virtue of spirals". When I read such statements, I groan inwardly. It is the force of gravity that drives water flow in rivers. By contrast, blood circulates in the human body apparently in defiance of gravity — and certainly not "by virtue of spirals". To equate the two phenomena is quite simply wrong — but then the Prince and his speechwriters are not ones to let an ugly fact get in the way of a beautiful metaphor.

There is, of course, nothing wrong with the future King of England not being well informed about the physiology of blood flow or any other medical technicality. But, discretion being the better part of valour, if he has only a tenuous grasp of a subject, it would surely behove him to refrain from commenting on it. Alternatively, he could solicit sound advice. Unfortunately, when it comes to alternative medicine, Prince Charles seems unable to do either.

If he had made just one factual blunder or merely expressed a passing interest in alternatives to standard medicine nobody would hold it against him. But Prince Charles rarely makes single lapses; indeed, his errors seem abundant, and his mis-statements are neither trivial nor irrelevant.

In his book, *Harmony: A New Way Of Looking At Our World*, he lectures us about human physiology and self-healing in a way which can only be described as embarrassing. He praises Taylor Still, the inventor of osteopathy, for being "empathic that disease was a disturbance in the natural flow of blood" and criticizes modern medicine for its "mechanistic view of the world". The truth is, of course, that Still's assumptions about the origins of disease being traceable to disturbed blood flow were both naïvely mechanistic and entirely groundless.

Reviewing Prince Charles's book, the journalist and historian Max Hastings wrote that the Prince "insists upon addressing a range of issues wider and deeper than any mortal man—unless he has the mind of a genius, as the Prince certainly does not—can sensibly encompass. Some of this book reads like the ravings of a Buddhist mystic". Hastings concluded: "Any-one who reads the Prince of Wales' new book will have little doubt that the chief peril to our royal institution in the decades ahead lies within his well-meaning, muddled, woolly head."

In 2004, the Prince used the occasion of a public lecture for health care professionals to inform his audience about the value of the Gerson diet, a starvation cancer diet usually combined with coffee enemas. The treatment is not supported by sound evidence of efficacy—on the contrary: it is a dangerous and cruel therapy that is more likely to hasten than to delay death. Yet Prince Charles openly expressed his conviction that the Gerson regimen cures cancer, even citing a case where, in his opinion, this has happened. Many cancer specialists and other health care professionals who, like me, were present at this lecture listened in slack jawed disbelief.

In an invited response published in the *British Medical Journal*, Professor Michael Baum, the leading British surgical oncologist and prolific cancer researcher, responded to the Prince's views: "The power of my authority comes with knowledge built on 40 years of study and 25 years of active involvement in cancer research. Your power and authority rests on an accident of birth. I don't begrudge you that authority but I do beg you to exercise your power with extreme caution when advising patients with life-threatening diseases to embrace unproven therapies."

Professor Baum knew whereof he spoke. He, too, had been a participant in the "Talking Health" colloquia mentioned above. At that time, he had criticized the "polite diplomacy" of the delegates regarding the overt nonsense that was being presented by Prince Charles:

> If I would stand up at a meeting of the Royal Geological Society and claim that the earth was flat, there would no doubt be members of the audience who would leap to their feet to refute such a suggestion... [yet] those present during the first two or three colloquia seemed to have been inhibited. My personal explanation for the cause of such inhibition is that none of us wish to see ourselves portrayed as reactionary stereotypes. Yet I am sure that on a number of occasions during the earlier colloquia we have felt like the little boy in Hans Christian Andersen's tale of the Emperor's New Clothes.

Possibly realizing that he had pushed the envelope too far and that some damage control might be needed, the Prince pretended to have been misunderstood about his promotion of the Gerson diet. According to a Clarence House spokesman, "The Prince of Wales is not promoting alternative medicines over orthodox treatments." But such hastily drawn up press releases are often demonstrably less than honest: in December 2000, Prince Charles himself had written in *NHS Magazine*: "...alternative medicine should be available to all on the NHS..."

While everyone is, of course, at liberty to use whatever nonsensical nostrums they choose, they should not expect to be able do so at the expense of their fellow citizens, nor should evidence-based treatments have to give way in order that scarce resources can be diverted to fund dangerous quackery.

Prince Charles seems to have an uncanny knack of selecting incompetent advisors. The late essayist Christopher Hitchens put it more succinctly than anyone else: "the heir to the throne seems to possess the ability to surround himself — perhaps by some mysterious ultramagnetic force? — with every moon-faced spoon-bender, shrub-flatterer, and water-diviner within range."

Christopher Hitchens also had a clear vision of the wider detrimental implications of such rampant irrationality and was keenly aware that attacks upon systematic thought are treason against civilization:

> Once the hard-won principles of reason and science have been discredited, the world will not pass into the hands of credulous herbivores who keep crystals by their sides and swoon over the poems of Khalil Gibran. The "vacuum" will be invaded instead by determined fundamentalists of every stripe who already know the truth by means of revelation and who actually seek real and serious power in the here and now. One thinks of the painstaking, cloud-dispelling labour of British scientists from Isaac Newton to Joseph Priestley to Charles Darwin to Ernest Rutherford to Alan Turing and Francis Crick, much of it built upon the shoulders of Galileo and Copernicus, only to see it causally slandered by a moral and intellectual weakling from the usurping House of Hanover.

In 2005, through his ill-fated "Foundation for Integrated Health", Prince Charles started an initiative to encourage NHS general practitioners to "offer a wide range of herbal and other alternative treatments to their patients". A spokesman for the Foundation said: "we believe that in time, by unifying like-minded doctors who want to integrate complementary health care into their practices, a wider range of treatments will be available to patients across the country."

Come again? "A wider range of treatments"?

The criterion for good health care is not the width or the range of available treatment choices but the careful balancing of potential risks of the options on offer against their anticipated benefits. Surely, the notion of choice is meaningless if what we are talking about is a choice between treatment options that are worthless or directly harmful.

***

A particular favourite of Prince Charles is homeopathy. In his book, *Harmony: A New Way Of Looking At Our World*, Charles responds to sceptics who insist that any perceived beneficial effect of homeopathy is due solely to a placebo response:

> It is for this reason that critics argue that it is a trick of the mind and that its remedies are nothing more than sugar pills. What none of those who take this view ever seem to acknowledge is that these remedies also work on animals, which are surely unlikely to be influenced by the placebo effect.

No doubt the Prince and the team of advisors working on his book thought they had sewn up the argument with this assertion. If so, they were wrong: the fact is that animals are just as prone to placebo effects as humans. Indeed, some of the most fundamental research on placebo responses was carried out in animals. The Russian physiologist Ivan Pavlov trained dogs by ringing a bell every time he fed them. He subsequently demonstrated that, after repeating this ritual for some time, he could get the animals' gastric juices flowing by just ringing the bell and without providing any food at all. Experts call this phenomenon "conditioning", and it is an integral part of the placebo response.

Furthermore, there is an abundance of research designed to test whether animals do, in fact, respond to homeopathic remedies differently than to placebos. The totality of this evidence closely mirrors what the research on human subjects reveals: the response to homeopathic remedies is indistinguishable from that to a placebo. If Prince Charles does not know any of that, so be it. If his advisors are ignorant of such rather fundamental facts, then the "painstaking, cloud-dispelling labour of British scientists", as Hitchens so aptly put it, has indeed been "casually slandered".

While I and my team in Exeter were trying our very best to evaluate alternative medicine scientifically, Prince Charles continued to make public statements concerning matters which he evidently did not truly comprehend, delivering opinions on things that he had not studied in sufficient depth and expounding on issues seemingly without paying heed to the opinions of those who had worked in the field and had a lifetime of experience behind them.

Some might concede that there nevertheless is an upside: everything the Prince says forces his opposition to sharpen their thinking in making their case to the public. But the dissemination of wrong information is not stimulating; wrong information is just wrong, and it is arguably even more wrong when delivered by someone to whom the public affords an exaggerated degree of deference based not on his superior knowledge, but solely on his class.

If Prince Charles were to engage in public discussions or debates with those who hold opposing views, it would at least allow a little transparency; people could then form a judgment based on the weight of the arguments presented. Interestingly, though, the Prince never ventures to have a public debate with anybody who disagrees with his odd ideas. In the best tradition of the old dogmatists, Prince Charles studiously evades anything that might expose or threaten his erroneous views.

The pinnacle of Prince Charles's career as a promoter of quackery came when, on 23 May 2006, he addressed the annual assembly of the World Health Organisation (WHO). Just as he did a quarter of a century earlier, when he delivered his speech to the BMA, he urged the delegates to start using unproven treatments routinely—this time on a global scale. Alternative therapies, he said, were not just good for minor ailments but also helpful for serious diseases like diabetes or heart disease. "We need to harness the best of modern science and technology, but not at the expense of losing the best of what complementary approaches have to offer. That is integrated health—it really is that simple."

No, Your Royal Highness, it is not that simple at all. We need to establish which treatments reproducibly generate more good than harm for the benefit of suffering patients. And that is not called "integrated health" but evidence-based medicine. Treating diabetes and heart disease with unproven therapies instead of evidence-based treatments on a global scale would, without a shadow of a doubt, cause the premature death of millions.

In health care, naïve assumptions have the potential to kill regardless of how well meaning they might be. The British writer and broadcaster Francis Wheen therefore described Prince Charles's address to the WHO as "barmy and pernicious". Integrated health care, he added, "means that unproven therapies should have the same status as evidence-based medicine". Lord Taverne, the Liberal Democrat peer and member of the House of Lords, went even further: "A democratic country cannot tolerate a monarch who meddles in political matters and whose views only command notice not because of expertise but because of a position that he owes solely to the accident of birth."

***

Prince Charles created his Foundation for Integrated Medicine in 1993, the same year I took up my chair at Exeter. The Foundation later changed its name to The Prince of Wales' Foundation for Integrated Health. Initially, there were occasional contacts between the Foundation and myself; I even served for a short while on one of its committees, the Foundation funded one of our studies of homeopathy, and they participated in several of our annual research meetings at Exeter. I would be lying, however, to say that the relationship between my team and the Foundation had ever been intense or warm. They appeared to be more interested in promoters than in scientists, and they seemed distinctly wary of even a hint of critical assessment.

Over the years I grew more and more suspicious of the Foundation's aims and, in parallel, the Foundation grew more and more dissatisfied with the results of my research and the public comments I increasingly made about alternative medicine. Rigorous science, it seemed, was only acceptable to them as long as the findings matched Prince Charles's expectations. The first tangible tensions emerged in 2005, when the Foundation published a document entitled *Complementary Healthcare: A Guide For Patients*.

This government-sponsored brochure informed patients about a range of alternative therapies using a standardized format with the following headings:

- What is the treatment commonly used for?

- What happens during a consultation?

- Precautions

- Cost

- Finding a practitioner

But where is the heading for "Effectiveness"? Anybody glancing through the booklet would quickly find that it lacked both critical input and hard evidence about the effectiveness of the included therapies. A patient guide without any discussion of the evidence underpinning a particular treatment, its potential risks and anticipated benefits surely contributes nothing to informed decision making. Imagine a government-sponsored patient guide on the use of painkillers that included no information whatsoever on how effective the most commonly used painkillers were, nor gave any hint about their risks or side effects. What good would such a booklet be? Yet the Foundation's guide contained none of these most basic facts and, when challenged about this omission, the Foundation argued that the Department of Health (DoH), which had commissioned the guide, had never asked for such information to be included.

I happen to have evidence, though, that this assertion is not correct.

A pre-publication draft of the guide had been sent to me for comment; it most definitely *did* include a summary of the evidence. As it contained numerous embarrassing mistakes, I offered to correct them. The offer was, however, rejected. Instead, the flawed evidence summary was simply erased, and the guide was published without it. Consequently, the guide merely "regurgitates proponent claims without indicating which are unsubstantiated and/or based on delusion", as HealthWatch put it at the time.

Because the guide seemed like a promotional brochure for quackery with the potential to cause considerable harm, I felt it was my moral and ethical duty to speak out. For the first time, I publicly opposed the Foundation, calling the guide "frankly inaccurate and over-optimistically misleading". Michael Fox, the Foundation's Chief Executive, then countered by claiming that "Professor Ernst's view has been fully taken into account", a statement which was demonstrably untrue.

The Foundation's press release claiming that the guide was "designed to help people choose a suitable therapy" seemed like a cynical joke. Deliberately withholding important information and thus depriving patients of the information necessary to make informed therapeutic decisions is not a trivial matter. The guide recommended chiropractic for digestive disorders, acupuncture for addictions and osteopathy for asthma — yet there is no scientific evidence whatsoever to support any of these recommendations. At the time, I called this "misleading" but, in hindsight, this term is actually far too kind; in fact, such unfounded claims even have the potential to cause the death of many patients. The Foundation's patient guide was nothing less than taxpayer-funded paean to quackery.

I remember thinking, how is it that I am the only expert to voice concern? Why are so many of my medical colleagues lending their tacit support to this ill-conceived and fundamentally deceptive document? Granted, I had precious few friends in the alternative medicine camp to start with but, after trying and failing to find answers to these questions, I discovered that I had even fewer friends — and considerably more enemies — than I had ever supposed. From here on, things only got worse.

***

The disagreement about the patient guide had been the first salvo in the dispute between Prince Charles, his sycophants and me. By contrast, the affair of the Smallwood Report led to a pitched battle in which my determination to be responsible and truthful about alternative medicine was ranged against what appeared to me as the Prince's attempts to slip alternative medicine quietly through the backdoor of the UK's National Health Service without the support of scientific evidence or the benefit of a full public debate.

It all started quite innocently. In March 2005, two friendly youngsters interviewed me; they worked for FreshMinds, a London-based commercial research consultancy that prides itself to be "a network of the sharpest analysts, consultants and researchers in Europe". My two visitors had made an appointment to see me in my offices and explained that the Prince of Wales' Foundation for Integrated Health had commissioned them to conduct a series of interviews with about a dozen leading UK experts in alternative medicine. The collection would then be published as a booklet and would inform public opinion on alternative medicine. The interview itself was uneventful, if not a bit dull, and the FreshMinds youngsters promised to send me the transcripts for final approval. Before they left, I recommended several other experts who took a critical stance toward alternative medicine, as I got the impression that they had lined up very little by way of critical input.

In July of the same year, the two FreshMinds interviewers visited me again, this time in the company of Christopher Smallwood, a retired economist who had previously worked for a major UK bank. The three visitors explained that, since their last visit, their remit had changed radically. The new aim, I was told, was to review the scientific evidence related to the cost-effectiveness of five popular forms of alternative medicine. This, I thought, was quite exciting: by total coincidence, I had just finished a project commissioned by the World Health Organisation with a very similar aim. Our review of all 27 economic evaluations available at the time had concluded that, due to the lack of rigour of these investigations, the question whether alternative medicine would save or cost extra money remained unanswered. As our report had already been accepted for publication, I tried to be as helpful as possible and offered an unpublished draft to my guests. To my surprise, they showed no interest at all in it. At this point, I began to feel slightly uncomfortable and couldn't help wondering what the real purpose of this appointment was.

My visitors elaborated that their cost-evaluation was to be supplemented with case studies and interviews, including the one I had previously given. The finished document, they explained, was to be handed directly to UK health ministers; crucially, there was not going to be any peer-review process or public debate. The goal of my guests and their report, it seemed to me, was to change UK health policy via a backdoor route. Realizing this, my alarm bells began to ring.

Mr Smallwood furthermore informed me that the report was no longer being commissioned via the Foundation; instead, the Prince of Wales had personally instructed him to do the research and write the report because he felt the Foundation was a "waste of space".

Exactly like the draft report, which I only saw *after* that meeting, the final report turned out to contain numerous factual errors and a wealth of misleading information, for instance:

- The report stated: "… a weekly course of St John's wort cost just 82p" and this expense, it was claimed, "compares well with the £13.82 for conventional antidepressants". This is incorrect. Using an appropriate dose of a high-quality extract such as the one that has been tested in clinical trials, the weekly cost for St John's wort in the UK would range from £8.40 to £16.80 — which is *not* cheaper than a conventional anti-depressant.

- Chondroitin, glucosamine and melatonin were listed as herbal medicines, which of course they are not: none of these supplements is plant-derived.

- Homeopathy was recommended as a cost-saving "alternative" for treating asthma, despite lack of evidence of efficacy.

- The widespread use of homeopathy, it was claimed, would save £4 billion on the national prescription drugs bill. Considering the published evidence from more than a dozen systematic reviews and meta-analyses, all of which failed to confirm that homeopathic remedies are more than a placebo, this was a shocking recommendation.

- And consider this: "…a number of alternative treatments offer the possibility of significant savings in direct health costs." The best available evidence certainly does not support this notion.

- Or this: "…there is a relatively large literature on the costs and benefits of homeopathy." At that time, and even today, there have been no rigorous UK studies on the issue at all.

- And this: "…if 4 per cent of GPs were to… [offer homeopathy]… a large saving (£190 million) would result." This, I felt, was not just cynically misleading, it was outright dangerous.

I was not the only one to be shocked. After the publication of the Smallwood Report, Richard Horton, editor of *The Lancet*, did not mince his words: "Let's be clear: this report contains dangerous nonsense."

During their visit to Exeter, both Mr Smallwood and the two FreshMinds interviewers had volunteered to me that they had no understanding of health care or of alternative medicine. Mr Smallwood even went so far as to argue that this was a positive thing, as it would protect him from accusations of bias.

When I finally did read the draft of the Smallwood Report I was truly dismayed. I immediately emailed Mr Smallwood, pointing out the many inaccuracies in the report and offering to correct them. However, my criticism did not go down well with the ex-economist. Our email exchanges became increasingly angry and eventually we agreed—not very politely, I should add—to disagree. At that point, I asked for my name to be removed from this embarrassingly flawed and dangerous document.

The battle-lines had been drawn, but it was not until several weeks later that open warfare broke out. In August 2005, a journalist from *The Times* telephoned me and asked whether I knew about the report, which at that point was about to be launched in the Houses of Parliament and handed over to health ministers. I answered that I had promised to keep the contents of the report confidential. Actually, I had given such a promise only in relation to the interview that took place between me and the two youngsters from FreshMinds on their first visit to my office. But even so, I told the journalist (whom I knew well and trusted implicitly) that I could not reveal the contents of the report to the press. He was not asking me to reveal any contents, he explained; the report had apparently already been leaked, and a copy lay before him on his desk as we were speaking. He simply wanted to know what my involvement had been, why I had withdrawn from the project and what I thought of the report's methodology, quality and reliability. So, after some hesitation, I decided to talk without disclosing any of the actual content of the report.

The next day I found my comments on the title page of *The Times*. In my excitement, I had voiced my opinions without equivocation. One remark seemed particularly crucial: "The Prince of Wales also seems to have overstepped his constitutional role." (A note to the reader: if you ever criticize Prince Charles, don't mention his rather frequent violations of his constitutional role. That seems to really upset him.)

On the same day, I received an email from Mr Smallwood which accused me of breaking my promise of confidentiality.

He also made an open threat that he would make my "transgressions" public "at an appropriate point". In fact, Smallwood wasted no time in mobilizing the "royal cavalry" in the shape of Prince Charles's first private secretary, Sir Michael Peat. On 22 September 2005, Peat wrote this letter on Clarence House notepaper to the Vice Chancellor of Exeter University:

> I am writing both as The Prince of Wales' Private Secretary and as Acting Chairman of His Royal Highness' Foundation for Integrated Health.
>
> There has been a breach of confidence by Professor Edzard Ernst in respect of a draft report on the efficacy of certain complementary therapies sent to him by Mr. Christopher Smallwood. The report was commissioned by The Prince of Wales.
>
> Mr. Smallwood sent Professor Ernst an early and, at that stage, incomplete draft of the report for comment. The accompanying e-mail requested and stressed the need for confidentiality. Professor Ernst implicitly agreed to comment on the report on this basis but then, as you probably saw, gave his views about the report to the national press. I attach a copy of a letter from the Editor of the *Lancet* published by *The Times* which summarises the issues well. I also attach a copy of the e-mail sent to Professor Ernst by Mr. Smallwood.
>
> I apologise for troubling you, but I felt that you should have this matter drawn to your attention.

What followed was the most unpleasant period of my entire professional life. Later I was told that, after receiving the letter, my Vice Chancellor had phoned Sir Michael Peat and asked him whether he really did want me investigated, as I might not take such a thing lying down. Peat's answer apparently had been affirmative.

The internal investigation into my alleged wrongdoing lasted 13 months, and during this time I was treated as guilty until proven innocent. There were several meetings during which I was interrogated, and dozens of cross-examining emails and letters. In the course of these actions, I had to take expensive legal advice, my quality of life went out the window, and even my health deteriorated.

With the help of my lawyers I formulated my defence along the following lines:

- I had not disclosed any contents of the report.

- I had only given a promise of confidentiality in relation to the initial FreshMinds interview study, but not in relation to Smallwood's bizarre cost-evaluation.

- As a doctor, researcher and UK citizen, I had an ethical and moral duty to prevent the considerable harm that the report was about to inflict on the British public.

- There was no opportunity for me — or anyone else — to submit criticisms of the report after publication, since it was specifically intended for delivery directly into the hands of health ministers and policymakers without the benefit of a public airing.

At the end of the investigation, on 13 October 2006, the Vice Chancellor wrote to me: "I have decided that it would not be appropriate to issue you with a formal disciplinary warning regarding this matter." Yet this grudging exoneration carried a sting in its tail: in the same letter, the Vice Chancellor made it clear that, in case I ever dared to do anything similar again, it "will certainly result in disciplinary action".

So there it was: I had been interrogated, investigated, treated like dirt for 13 months and exonerated in the end. But even while acknowledging that I had not been guilty of any mis-demeanour, my Vice Chancellor had issued an unambiguous warning to me: if I even thought of applying my personal ethical standards in any similar situation in the future, I would not be so lucky as to get away with it again.

Prince Charles's attempt to silence me, it seemed, had been successful.

Well, perhaps not. Had the Vice Chancellor known me better, had he ever even once discussed these matters with me in person, he could have saved himself from the ridicule that resulted from his threat of future disciplinary action. Since receiving his shameful letter, I have spoken out on many further occasions, and I fully intend to continue doing so. If anything, his sabre-rattling made me even more determined to fight quackery, regardless of whether or not the quack in question happened to be a member of the House of Windsor.

In March 2007, ITV aired a programme entitled "The Meddling Prince" in which the Smallwood Report case was featured prominently.[1] After this, politicians, scientists and other prominent figures began rallying to my support. This put Prince Charles and his courtiers in an embarrassing position. The reaction of Clarence House was remarkable for its duplici-tousness. Sir Michael Peat, who evidently had written the formal complaint on Clarence House notepaper, now declared: "This letter was not prompted by His Royal Highness and he was not even aware that it had been written." Yet, the first sentence of that very letter ("I am writing as the Prince of Wales' Principal Private Secretary…") suggested otherwise. Mean-while, the unrepentant Christopher Smallwood continued to hurl the same exhaustively discredited accusation, calling me "thoroughly disreputable" and publicly commenting: "to go to the papers after his undertaking to me was the most blatant and disreputable breach of confidence I have ever known."

Being investigated by the very university administration that should have most strenuously defended and supported me was, of course, profoundly disappointing. But a much more important consequence of the Smallwood story had yet to reveal itself.

The University had signed a contract committing to raising £1.5 million for my unit. After the intervention by Clarence House, all fundraising activities abruptly stopped. As a result, our funds were gradually exhausted. In 2011, the Vice Chan-

---

1   The programme, or at least part of it, can still be seen: http://
     www.dailymotion.com/video/x1k00d_charles-the-meddling-prince-
     part-2_tech.

cellor decided to close my unit. The survival of the only research team worldwide that had been steadfastly devoted to the critical evaluation of alternative medicine was therefore imperilled.

***

My job was to scientifically assess alternative medicine. That position carried with it a duty to warn the public of dangerous quackery and health fraud. This remit had been established from the outset, and had been codified in the explicit wording of the mission statement that I had laid down in the earliest days of my tenure at Exeter. I saw no reason whatever to change my scientific goals or my research strategy, no matter who decided to threaten me.

The year 2009 marked a new apogee in Prince Charles's accelerating promotion of quackery, when Duchy Originals, the retail firm that he had founded in 1990, signed an agreement with several upscale food stores in the UK to market a new line of herbal remedies to the unsuspecting public.

Duchy Originals claimed that their "Detox Tincture", containing extracts of dandelion and artichoke, could eliminate poisons from the body. Of course, this is utter nonsense: neither ingredient is capable of eliminating toxins — besides, the entire notion of detoxification as used and promoted in alternative medicine is biologically meaningless and confers absolutely no health benefits. Furthermore, at £10 per 50ml, this tincture was expensive. This, coupled with the blatantly false claims being made for this product, seemed to me to represent unvarnished quackery.

There are, of course, many other bogus detox products. But this one was different; it stood out because it was produced and promoted by the Prince's firm, Duchy Originals. Thus it enjoyed a distinct marketing advantage: with Prince Charles as its figurehead and his royal imprimatur, its public impact was likely to be considerably stronger than any other detox product available at that time.

Once again I decided to go public, dubbing his potions "dodgy originals" and stating: "Charles financially exploits a gullible public in a time of financial hardship." And once again I was reprimanded.

When the Dean, Prof John Tooke, ordered me to his office, I had little doubt as to the reason for the summons. Luckily — and entirely without my instigation or participation — by the time the appointment took place the UK regulatory authorities had already ruled that the advertising for the Duchy Originals herbal tinctures was not in compliance with the law. The manufacturer was compelled to change it — a regulatory showdown that did not escape the press. Consequently, when we met, Dean Tooke knew he no longer had a leg to stand on, and the anticipated reprimand turned out to be a sheepish "do you always have to be so undiplomatic?" type of discussion.

***

To mark the occasion of my retirement from Exeter, in May 2011, the London-based Science Media Centre, an institution that aims to facilitate the dialogue between scientists and the press, invited me to give a press conference. This organization had long had an interest in my research, and its boss, Fiona Fox, had repeatedly asked me to attend their meetings and present my results to a small, hand-picked group of journalists. Now Fiona felt that my retirement would be a good opportunity to review my two decades of investigating alternative medicine.

Contrary to many scientists, I have always enjoyed a good working relationship with journalists. I had realized some time ago that journalists had a most important role to play in disseminating accurate information about medicine, particularly its alternative variety. The average consumer frequently does not seek advice from health care professionals about alternative medicine but instead relies on what s/he reads in the papers or online. This makes it doubly important that journalists report the facts correctly and responsibly. Based on this reasoning, I had forged several reliable links with journalists from the UK and abroad who knew they could turn to me to verify facts or summarize the evidence concerning this or that alternative treatment.

With this background, I looked forward to my presentation at the Science Media Centre and had prepared what I hoped would be an entertaining 15-minute lecture. In it, I had stressed several arguments that had been important themes of my research. One such theme was that of the current ubiquity of snake-oil salesmen. This is, of course, absolutely true: during the previous two decades, my team could hardly conduct research fast enough to keep up with the endless flow of irresponsible claims being made by ruthless entrepreneurs for alternative therapies.

During my lecture, I briefly mentioned the story of the Duchy Originals Detox Tincture as a case in point. I did this to stress another important issue, namely that science alone is frequently inadequate to the task of keeping the public informed about the dangers of quackery. I had, of course, published many articles in medical journals about the fact that detoxification as used in alternative medicine had no plausible basis and was not backed up by any evidence. Yet the existence of articles in medical journals seemed to have insufficient influence to prevent the public from falling victim to bogus claims. My theory, which I put to the journalists, was that responsible, well-informed journalism had a crucial role to play in encouraging critical thinking, particularly on the subject of alternative medicine.

My lecture was well received and, during question time, the journalist from *The Daily Mail* swiftly linked my two themes by asking, "Would you say that Prince Charles is a snake-oil salesman?" I answered the only way I could: "Yes."

The next day, virtually all the UK national papers carried the story. *The Daily Mail* ran it with the title "Charles? He's just a snake-oil salesman…" The text explained:

> Prince Charles has been branded a "snake-oil salesman" by Britain's first professor of complementary medicine for supporting "dodgy" alternative therapies. Professor Edzard Ernst claimed yesterday that the prince's backing for "unproven and disproven" remedies was an attempt to smuggle them into the NHS despite scientific evidence showing they could be dangerous.

***

From my perspective, the story of Prince Charles's keen interest in alternative medicine is foremost a story of missed opportunities. Everyone seems to agree that he is full of good intentions; he undoubtedly has influence and therefore the ability to raise funds and generate progress. The fact that he has used his uniquely privileged position to hinder scientific research while actively promoting quackery is, I think, a tragic waste.

I had long been aware of the risks of entering into open conflict with somebody as elevated as Prince Charles. On the one hand, it was always clear to me that I had much to lose in such a fight. On the other hand, there were important issues at stake: truth, honesty, progress and patient safety, to mention just a few. Most importantly, I had to abide by my own scientific, moral and ethical standards. In the final analysis, I simply did not have a choice: I had to do what I was sure was right.

And come to think of it, I would do it all over again if I had to.

Chapter 8

The End of the Road

During my professional career I have been on the faculty of five different universities and have been appointed to full professorships in Germany, Austria and Britain as well as visiting professorships in the US and Canada. If this experience has taught me anything, it is that the world of academia is not always the comfortably sheltered environment that it is so often made out to be.

After my time in Vienna, where I experienced more than my fair share of intrigue and machination, I had sincerely hoped that Exeter would be a little more peaceful. And, initially at least, it turned out very much that way. At the medical school in Vienna there had been about four hundred professors, and we were all expected to sit on countless committees. By contrast, at the time I joined the faculty in Exeter, its postgraduate medical school could boast a grand total of three professors. Consequently, life there was agreeably quiet. But in 2000, when the Peninsula Medical School was established, this situation began to change.

When John Tooke became the new Dean of the Peninsula Medical School we had been friends for some years, and I was confident that, in his new position, he would become a useful ally and staunch supporter of my research. From previous encounters, I had gained the impression that, although he did not perceive alternative medicine as a subject worthy of serious consideration, he was nevertheless impressed by our publication record, and by the national profile and international reputation my team was beginning to enjoy. These things do count for a lot in academia and are important for any medical school, especially so for a brand-new one.

At four-yearly intervals, all UK academic institutions must undergo what is known as the Research Assessment Exercise, a review process designed to evaluate the quality of research being done at those institutions with the aim of deciding on the apportionment of public funds to support research during the next four years. While some researchers at Exeter had a hard time marshalling enough high quality research articles for submission, the problem faced by my unit consisted more in deciding which of our numerous publications we should submit: our publication rate in top medical journals was second to none.

Any medical school depends to a very large extent on funding from government, charities and private donors, so the public image of our school, and in particular the way it is depicted in the national press, is of considerable importance. It was therefore predictable, perhaps, that this would be the subject on which Tooke and I had our first real differences of opinion.

Aware that my unit attracted much more press interest than any other department of "his" new medical school, and feeling somewhat nervous about the unvarnished frankness with which I often talked to journalists, the Dean notified me that my contacts with the press would henceforth have to be limited, and that he wanted to "be informed about PR activities", as he put it in an email.

What followed was a somewhat unsettling correspondence between us in which he expressed views that seemed to me to be inconsistent with the principles of academic freedom and free speech. Essentially, he wanted to control what I said to journalists. For my part, I felt that it was up to me to decide how I responded to enquiries from the press regarding my research (I never approached journalists on my own initiative). Eventually, he put an end to the discussion by declaring that his decision was non-negotiable: henceforth I was to obtain permission for what he termed "every major" exchange involving the press. This seemed the academic equivalent of a D notice: either I cut myself off voluntarily from all contacts with the press, or Tooke would step in and act as gatekeeper, allowing me to speak to journalists only on those topics that he considered appropriate and not politically sensitive.

Faced with this ultimatum I had little choice. I managed to continue responding to enquiries from the press for a while longer by interpreting his definition of "major" as broadly as possible. Inevitably, though, this led to further disagreements: press coverage of a positive story (e.g. "professor finds that acupuncture is safe") would usually pass without comment, while negative news (e.g. "professor finds that homeopathy does not work") would promptly elicit a reprimand.

Of course, this atmosphere, tense and heavy with implicit — and increasingly explicit — hostility, could not continue indefinitely. The watershed came in 2003, when I saw an announcement published in the newsletter of the Prince of Wales' Foundation for Integrated Health:

> The Peninsula Medical School aims to become the UK's first medical school to include integrated medicine at postgraduate level. The school also plans to extend the current range and depth of programmes offered by including healthcare ethics and legislation. Professor John Tooke, dean of the Peninsula Medical School, said: "The inclusion of integrated medicine is a patient driven development. Increasingly the public is turning to the medical profession for information about complementary medicines. This programme will play an important role in developing critical understanding of a wide range of therapies".

When I stumbled on this announcement, I was truly puzzled. Tooke is obviously planning a new course for me, I thought, but why has he not told me about it? When I enquired, Tooke informed me that the medical school was indeed preparing to offer a postgraduate "Pathway in Integrated Health"; this exciting new innovation had been initiated by Dr Michael Dixon, a general practitioner who, after working in collaboration with my unit for several years, had become one of the UK's most outspoken proponents of spiritual healing and other similarly dubious forms of alternative medicine. For this reason, Dixon was apparently very well regarded by Prince Charles.

A few days after I had received this amazing news, Dixon arrived at my office and explained, with visible embarrassment, that Prince Charles had expressed his desire to him personally to establish such a course at Exeter. His Royal Highness had already facilitated its funding which, in fact, came from "Nelsons", one of the UK's largest manufacturers of homeopathic remedies. The day-to-day running of the course was to be put into the hands of the ex-director of the Centre for Complementary Health Studies (CCHS), the very unit that, almost a decade earlier, I had struggled—and eventually even paid—to be separated from because of its overtly anti-scientific agenda. The whole thing had been in the planning for many months. I was, it seemed, the last to know—but now that I had learnt about it, Dixon and Tooke leaned on me with all their might to persuade me to contribute to this course by giving a few lectures.

I could no more comply with this request than fly. Apart from anything else, anyone who had read my papers would have known that I was opposed in principle to the concept of "Integrated Health". As I saw it, "integrating" quackery with genuine, science-based medicine was nothing less than a profound betrayal of the ethical basis of medical practice. By putting its imprimatur on this course, and by offering it under the auspices of a mainstream medical school, my institution would be encouraging the dangerously erroneous idea of equivalence—i.e. the notion that alternative and mainstream medicine were merely two parallel but equally valid and effective methods of treating illness.

To add insult to injury, the course was to be run by someone who I had good reason to reject and sponsored by a major manufacturer of homeopathic remedies. In all conscience, the latter circumstance seemed to me to be the last straw. Study after study carried out by my unit had found homeopathy to be not only conceptually absurd but also therapeutically worthless. To all intents and purposes, the discussion about the value of homeopathy was closed. Even a former director of the Royal London Homeopathic Hospital had concluded in his book that "homeopathy has not been proved to work... the great majority... of the improvement that patients experience is due to non-specific causes". If we did not take a stand on this issue, we might as well give up and go home. Consequently, I politely but firmly declined the offer of participating in this course.

By now numerous other incidents of a similar nature had poisoned the atmosphere at my own medical school and university so much that both my work and my health were suffering. How had it come to this? Why was even the most obvious and demonstrable truth being turned upside down so that it could be used against me? Why were my peers seemingly bent on constraining me and making life increasingly difficult for me?

This was by no means a trivial question and, on reflection, the most plausible answer, in my view, was that the results of my research were a thorn in the flesh of powerful interests operating in the background. Our critical analyses of alternative medicine, once acclaimed locally, nationally and internationally, seemed no longer wanted.

It was time to take a step back, talk things over with Danielle and assess the situation as objectively as I could. For more than a decade, I had done precisely the job that the University had hired me to do. I had worked extremely hard to establish an outstanding international reputation for our unit, with obvious benefits to the medical school and the University. On several occasions I had been told "you have put Exeter on the academic map". This might just have been flattery, but surely nobody could dispute that we had done amazingly well. For the first years that the new medical school had been in existence, my team had published more papers in the peer-reviewed medical literature than the rest of that institution put together. Even today, there is not a single academic in the whole of Exeter University who has published more in the last two decades than I have. My "H-Index", a widely used measure to quantify an academic's standing, was around 80, more than twice that of any other faculty member of the medical school. These facts alone should have earned me the appreciation of my institution.

Was I being unreasonable? Were the obstacles and problems I was increasingly encountering just the normal "rough and tumble" any academic researcher might come across? I considered this possibility seriously but it simply couldn't account for the way things had so clearly and dramatically changed. Virtually all the financial, administrative and moral support I once had enjoyed had disappeared; my team and I were systematically isolated; the importance of our work was constantly belittled; and I was made to feel that my hard work was not an asset but a burden to the University. Anyone visiting the medical school could have been forgiven for thinking that my unit did not even exist. A glossy brochure describing the research activities of the Peninsula Medical School, for instance, altogether failed to mention us—and that was at a time when we were authoring more papers than the rest of the school put together.

There seemed to be very little I could do to improve the situation. Of course, if I had been prepared to change the direction or attitude of my research and become more "politically correct", I might have ingratiated myself with the Dean, the Vice Chancellor and all the others who were so visibly irritated by me. Virtually all research groups in alternative medicine were conducting an entirely different kind of science, so why couldn't we?

The easiest way to study alternative medicine in the "politically correct" way would have been to investigate how many patients use it, to monitor how satisfied users of alternative medicine were, to evaluate why some people preferred alternative to conventional therapies, and so on. Invariably, the results would then show that this sector of health care is surprisingly popular, and from that one could then comfortably and non-controversially conclude that, "if people use it, are satisfied with it, and even pay for it, alternative medicine must be good." This line of enquiry would not rock anyone's boat and would make everyone—including Prince Charles—happy. But, as I see it, this type of research is irrelevant, inconsequential and intrinsically misleading. Certainly it is not what I ever considered to be rigorous, high-quality science and most definitely it would not have been in line with our mission statement. To change direction in this way was not a reasonable option, at least not for me. I was not prepared to sacrifice my integrity as a scientist for the sake of avoiding being given a rough ride by those who opposed me and were disquieted by my research findings.

But what should I do? The future of my entire team depended on the answer to this question. After many sleepless nights and several anxious meetings with the team, together we decided to batten down the hatches, try to be as self-sufficient as possible, and simply get on with our job as before. Aggrieved though we felt, we did not look for praise; we did not need a red carpet to be rolled out for us; we merely wished to be treated fairly and be left in peace to conduct our research.

Try as we might, though, the worsening tension and the frigid to hostile collegial atmosphere inevitably had a significant impact. The team slowly began to disintegrate: our morale, work ethic and enthusiasm seemed to be ebbing away. I had been so very proud of the group that I assembled and held together, a team of highly motivated, skilled, loyal and industrious researchers with whom I had worked closely for almost 15 years. Now it was becoming impossible to sustain these high standards when, at almost every one of our weekly staff meetings, we were forced to discuss the glaring lack of support and the overtly obstructive behaviour we had to contend with.

Inevitably, these problems also took a personal toll. For the first time in my life I became a regular visitor to my GP. To my dismay, within the space of just a few months, I had developed three different stress-related illnesses. The situation was not only making my work more and more difficult, it was progressively robbing me of my health.

Amidst these professional and personal difficulties, I decided to explore one last, desperate attempt to save my unit,

and with it the important work of continuing a critical evaluation of alternative medicine.

As my own salary was the largest of my team, I considered
cutting my working hours and taking half pay so that that Sir
Maurice's endowment could be made to last longer. I enquired
whether this was an option and asked my administration to
calculate the impact and outline the feasibility of prolonging the
life of my unit in this way. My hope was that my right hand
man and deputy, Dr Max Pittler, could ease into my shoes and
eventually take over from me entirely, allowing me to retire
early. Perhaps a new leadership could open the door to a fresh
start, new prospects and even a renewed source of funding.

Unfortunately the administration was unable—or
unwilling?—to discuss with me what financial consequences
my semi-retirement would have. This, along with many other
indicators, strongly suggested that neither the University nor
the medical school were at all interested in securing the long-
term future of our research unit.

In this situation, it was everyone for him- or herself. My co-
workers obviously had first and foremost to look after their own
employment and career prospects. Dr Pittler decided to take up
the post of research director at the German equivalent of the
National Institute for Clinical Excellence (NICE). On the one
hand, this was a strong testament to our achievements in
research: after all, Pittler had joined us straight after medical
school, and everything he had achieved was due to our
collective efforts. On the other hand, his decision to leave
seemed in a potent but unspoken way to seal the fate of our
unit.

Although the University had long ago signed a legally
binding contract committing to raising £1.5 million towards our
research, there was no sign of any effort to follow through on
that obligation. Indeed, it seemed to me that my peers had
quietly agreed amongst themselves to switch off my unit's life
support and were now simply biding their time, waiting for me
to take the hint and cooperate by exiting. When I failed to
oblige, Tooke declared that, due to lack of funds, it had been

decided that my unit would be closed down, all my staff would be dismissed or relocated, and I would have to take early retirement.

So there it was at last: my research team had been disbanded.[1]

For almost two decades my professional life and my whole identity had been inextricably bound up with the work of my unit. I had gone to Exeter with high hopes, confident that I was entering an institution wholeheartedly dedicated to the pursuit of high quality scientific enquiry. Instead I had to realize that, under certain circumstances, science could be perceived as an unwelcome intrusion.

Lawyer friends urged me earnestly to take the university to court; they were convinced that I would win. However, I had reached the end of the road. After so many years of feuding, I was bone weary and had no wish to become embroiled in protracted legal proceedings.

It was time to go.

---

[1]   After John Tooke had left Exeter, the new dean seemed to have a more open and sympathetic attitude towards my position. He and I agreed that I would volunteer to take early retirement and, in return, he would try to save my unit from closing. He even offered to re-employ me on a half-time basis after my official retirement in order to help him find a successor. Unfortunately, though, a suitable successor was never identified, nor were any funds made available for that post.

Coda

After publishing *Trick or Treatment* with Simon Singh in 2008, it dawned on me that certain aspects of my experience as a researcher of alternative medicine might be of interest to the wider public. This was when I began work on this book. Those who read early drafts strongly advised me to widen the focus and to include not just my "Exeter years" but also those that had come before. This effectively turned the book into a memoir and a much more personal account than I had originally wanted.

Looking back to my childhood, I see a timid boy who grew into a somewhat rebellious adolescent, frequently challenging his elders and asking uncomfortable questions. I am not sure I have changed that much since then. Certainly a tendency towards doubt and irreverence, coupled with an irrepressible sense of curiosity, have remained prominent features of my character and were doubtlessly influential in leading me towards becoming a scientist tackling awkward subjects.

At first glance, the two topics of my research during recent decades—alternative medicine and health care during the Third Reich—might appear to be almost entirely unrelated. On closer inspection, however, intriguing links on several levels do emerge.

Alternative medicine was embraced enthusiastically by the Nazis. They called it *Naturheilkunde* (natural medicine), and its integration with conventional health care under the banner of *Neue Deutsche Heilkunde* (New German Medicine) became an officially sanctioned health policy early on during the Third

Reich. With its emphasis on inexpensive, natural and whole-some treatments, alternative medicine appealed to the National Socialist worldview, in which the acquisition of optimum health was seen as a patriotic duty of the German *Volk* and a moral virtue befitting the supposedly superior Aryan race.

The Nazi policy of deliberately amalgamating alternative and conventional medicine bears many similarities to what is today known as "integrative medicine". The Nazis also created an entirely new health profession of non-medically trained practitioners of alternative medicine—the *Heilpraktiker*—a profession which is still very much in existence. Similarly, the influence of Nazi theories concerning "natural health" can also be seen in the contemporary school of alternative medicine known as *Germanische Neue Medizin* (German New Medicine), which promotes itself as a method of curing all sorts of conditions, including cancer. It is the bizarre brainchild of a German physician who seems to think that mainstream medi-cine is a Jewish conspiracy whose sole purpose is to annihilate gentiles.

Apologists for alternative medicine do not like reading this sort of information and tend to get upset by it. In 2013, Peter Fisher, the Queen's homeopath and editor of the journal *Homeo-pathy*, even fired me from the editorial board of his journal stating that I had "smeared homeopathy and other forms of complementary medicine with a 'guilt by association' argu-ment, associating them with the Nazis". But the association between alternative medicine and the Third Reich is surely not my invention; it is an indisputable historical fact, and nothing can be gained by ignoring it.

From a personal perspective, the most enduring impact of my investigations into this dark period of modern European history was a growing awareness of the overriding importance of medical ethics. My research into the Nazis' violations of medical ethics and their deliberate use of pseudoscience in pursuit of ideological ends had sensitized me and sent a clear signal: once we lose our focus on the basic principles that must govern medicine at all times, health care professionals can, and often do, behave atrociously.

A rather dramatic reminder of the link between Nazi ideology and alternative medicine was provided by the unlikely figure of Claus Fritzsche, a German journalist who regularly published pro-quackery essays for the unsuspecting German public and had long used this platform to systematically defame me. This did not bother me all that much; I had, after all, grown used to vitriolic attacks from promoters of pseudoscience. But Fritzsche's pillorying took a more sinister complexion when it was revealed in the *Süddeutsche Zeitung* that he was being paid generously by several large German manufacturers of homeopathic remedies to publish his defamatory articles. Intrigued, I decided to research Fritzsche's activities in more depth and, in doing so, I stumbled upon an entirely unexpected nexus between my two major research themes.

On 1 May 1945, just after Hitler had taken his life, Magda and Josef Goebbels (Reich Minister of Propaganda) killed themselves and six of their children in Hitler's Berlin bunker. The only child of the Goebbels family to survive was Harald Quandt, Magda's son from her first marriage, whom Goebbels had adopted. After the war, Quandt turned industrialist and became the owner of several large enterprises, including a leading homeopathic manufacturer. This company turned out to be one of those paying Fritzsche to write his derogatory articles. After the *Süddeutsche Zeitung* had disclosed these financial arrangements, the companies ended their financial support of Fritzsche. On 14 January 2014, about two years after these events, Fritzsche took his own life.

This depressing story speaks for itself and confirms something that I had become sure of: the most important link between my research into alternative medicine and that related to the Third Reich was that of medical ethics.

It should be axiomatic that ethics is indispensable to the practice of medicine, and is not something that can just be switched off at will. No branch of health care, including alternative medicine, can be considered exempt from it. But the subject of ethics is seldom even considered in alternative medicine; many alternative practitioners have never been taught medical ethics, and where training in this area does exist, it tends to be at best superficial. There are thousands of books on alternative medicine but hardly more than a handful cover the subject of medical ethics in any depth. It is perhaps not surprising, therefore, that the principles of medical ethics are routinely ignored and frequently violated by promoters of alternative medicine.

Medical ethics seem to me to be violated, for example: when homeopaths prescribe or recommend homeopathic vaccinations for which there is not a shred of evidence; when chiropractors or other alternative practitioners happily promote bogus treatments for children with asthma or other serious conditions; when practitioners fail to obtain informed consent before commencing their treatments; when Prince Charles sells his "detox tincture" which is unable to eliminate poisons from your body, merely cash from your purse; when quacks inveigle desperate cancer patients by pretending they have found a cure; when pharmacists sell Bach Flower Remedies or other glorified placebos; when applied kinesiologists, iridologists, etc. claim that their baseless diagnostic tests are able to identify serious diseases; when pseudoscientists claim that certain alternative therapies are evidence-based because they managed to generate a false positive result purely by cherry-picking or massaging their data; when politicians who lack even the most basic understanding of science publicly support quackery, proclaiming that it is evidence-based.

And so on, and so on.

Some might criticize me here for claiming the moral high ground. But if I do so, it is for a good reason. Medical consultations are intrinsically unequal, with the clinician occupying a position of considerable power over often highly vulnerable patients. This places an important ethical onus on the caregiver to assist patients in making informed choices—an imperative and a trust that is breached each and every time that unproven nostrums born of ideology and wishful thinking are offered to people with assertions that they are an effective, valid approach to the treatment of disease.

When science is abused, hijacked or distorted in order to serve political or ideological belief systems, ethical standards will inevitably slip. The resulting pseudoscience is a deceit perpetrated on the weak and the vulnerable. We owe it to ourselves, and to those who come after us, to stand up for the truth, no matter how much trouble this might bring.

Today, I look back at the often stormy past from the peaceful vantage point of my retirement with a mixture of satisfaction and incredulity. The doctor and scientist may still be full of questions, but the musician in me breathes a sigh of relief that the performance, with all its impossible demands and fiendishly difficult passages, is finally over.

Addendum

It is not my intention here to give a complete and detailed account of all our publications and findings. Yet a very brief summary of some of the most important conclusions reached during two decades of research into alternative medicine might be helpful.

<u>Acupuncture</u> was at the centre of our research from the very beginning. Our investigations suggest that it might be useful for certain conditions, particularly for some types of pain, and for alleviating nausea. Our research also shows that acupuncture relies to a large degree on the placebo effect. Whether acupuncture is truly effective beyond placebo is currently still unclear. More clinical trials comparing acupuncture with an adequate placebo (such as our 'stage-dagger' retracting needle) might eventually provide a conclusive answer.

As to the safety of acupuncture, we have demonstrated that, in the hands of adequately trained therapists, it rarely causes serious problems. In countries where acupuncturists are not well-educated, caution is advised because of the risk of cross-infection or injury to internal organs.

<u>Chiropractic</u> or osteopathic spinal manipulation might well be useful for back- and neck pain. However, even for these symptoms, it does not seem to be better than other treatments such as physiotherapeutic exercises or massage therapy. Considering its risks and costs, it is likely that spinal manipulation is less useful than conventional therapies.

There is currently no good evidence that spinal manipulation is effective for non-spinal conditions. It is thus high time that chiropractors and osteopaths desist from misleading the public with bogus therapeutic claims about the general health benefits of spinal manipulation or mobilization.

There is no doubt that mild to moderate adverse effects are very frequent. Whether and how frequently serious complications like strokes and deaths are caused by neck manipulation is less clear and is often hotly debated. My view is that, until we are sure, it is wise to be cautious.

Herbal medicine is an area where we find some of the best evidence in all of alternative medicine. Some herbal extracts contain pharmacologically active compounds that obviously can have health effects — both positive and negative. This means that some herbal supplements are effective but the question is, which? In the absence of regulatory oversight to enforce standards for purity, concentration and dosage limits, herbal medicines may very definitely cause harm. As there are thousands of different medicinal herbs, it is impossible to provide general judgments about the value of herbal medicines. It would therefore seem prudent to be careful; the best general advice is probably to rely on sound evidence either from a responsible, qualified practitioner with a sound grasp of pharmacognosy, or a well-researched, scientifically accurate text.

Traditional herbalists usually individualize their treatments according to the unique characteristics of each patient, an approach that seems very attractive to many patients. Unfortunately the evidence fails to show that such personalization generates more good than harm. This little known fact is, I think, important: in most countries, it is this type of herbalism that patients are exposed to when they consult a practitioner. In other words, the most commonly used approach in herbal medicine is not evidence-based and has the potential to cause considerable harm.

<u>Massage therapy</u> remains relatively under-researched, and therefore it is difficult to arrive at firm judgments about its usefulness. Fortunately it causes very few problems. On balance, the evidence does indicate that massage therapy can have relaxing effects. Through this mechanism, massage can alleviate a wide range of symptoms from anxiety to musculo-skeletal pain.

<u>Homeopathy</u> is one of the least plausible treatments in the realm of alternative medicine. The clinical evidence, both for humans and animals, even though not entirely uniform, does not suggest that homeopathic remedies have effects beyond those of placebos. In 2014, after conducting the most comprehensive and independent review of homeopathy to date, the Australian National Health and Medical Research Council put it more succinctly than most: "the evidence from research in humans does not show that homeopathy is effective for treating the range of [68] health conditions considered."

Contrary to what we are often told, the risks of homeopathy can be considerable. When someone chooses to embrace an ineffective treatment instead of pursuing effective therapy for a serious condition, even seemingly innocent remedies can, by default, turn out to be life-threatening.

AKNOWLEDGEMENTS: Throughout my life, I have benefitted enormously from the support of family, friends, co-workers and peers. The list is far too long to be printed here, but I want to thank them all nevertheless.

Special thanks, however, goes to Louise Lubetkin who helped me immeasurably with this book at a time when I had almost given up hope of ever publishing it.